Occupational Asthma

Guest Editor

DAVID I. BERNSTEIN, MD

IMMUNOLOGY AND ALLERGY CLINICS OF NORTH AMERICA

www.immunology.theclinics.com

Consulting Editor
RAFEUL ALAM, MD, PhD

November 2011 • Volume 31 • Number 4

SAUNDERS an imprint of ELSEVIER, Inc.

W.B. SAUNDERS COMPANY

A Division of Elsevier Inc.

1600 John F. Kennedy Blvd., • Suite 1800 • Philadelphia, PA 19103-2899.

http://www.theclinics.com

IMMUNOLOGY AND ALLERGY CLINICS OF NORTH AMERICA Volume 31, Number 4

November 2011 ISSN 0889–8561, ISBN-13: 978-1-4557-1104-8

Editor: Rachel Glover
Developmental Editor: Donald Mumford

Immunology and Allergy Clinics of North America (ISSN 0889–8561) is published quarterly by Elsevier Inc., 360 Park Avenue South, New York, NY 10010-1710. Months of issue are February, May, August, and November. Periodicals postage paid at New York, NY and additional mailing offices. Subscription prices are $272.00 per year for US individuals, $392.00 per year for US institutions, $129.00 per year for US students and residents, $334.00 per year for Canadian individuals, $187.00 per year for Canadian students, $486.00 per year for Canadian institutions, $379.00 per year for international individuals, $486.00 per year for international institutions, $187.00 per year for international students. To receive student/resident rate, orders must be accompanied by name of affiliated institution, date of term, and the *signature* of program/residency coordinator on institution letterhead. Orders will be billed at individual rate until proof of status is received. Foreign air speed delivery is included in all *Clinics* subscription prices. All prices are subject to change without notice. **POSTMASTER**: Send address changes to *Immunology and Allergy Clinics of North America*, Elsevier Health Sciences Division, Subscription Customer Service, 3251 Riverport Lane, Maryland Heights, MO 63043. **Customer Service:** 1-800-654-2452 (U.S. and Canada); 314-447-8871 (outside U.S. and Canada). Fax: 314-447-8029. E-mail: journalscustomerservice-usa@elsevier.com(for print support); journalsonlinesupport-usa@elsevier.com (for online support).

Reprints. For copies of 100 or more, of articles in this publication, please contact the Commercial Reprints Department, Elsevier Inc., 360 Park Avenue South, New York, New York 10010-1710. Tel. (212) 633-3812, Fax: (212) 462-1935, e-mail: reprints@elsevier.com.

Immunology and Allergy Clinics of North America is covered in MEDLINE/PubMed (Index Medicus), Current Contents/Life Sciences, Science Citation Index, ISI/BIOMED, Chemical Abstracts, and EMBASE/Excerpta Medica.

Printed and bound by CPI Group (UK) Ltd, Croydon, CR0 4YY

Transferred to Digital Print 2011

Contributors

CONSULTING EDITOR

RAFEUL ALAM, MD, PhD
Veda and Chauncey Ritter Chair in Immunology, Professor, and Director, Division of Immunology and Allergy, National Jewish Health; and University of Colorado Health Sciences Center, Denver, Colorado

GUEST EDITOR

DAVID I. BERNSTEIN, MD
Professor of Medicine and Environmental Health, Division of Immunology, Allergy and Rheumatology, University of Cincinnati College of Medicine, Cincinnati, Ohio

AUTHORS

DAVID I. BERNSTEIN, MD
Professor of Medicine and Environmental Health, Division of Immunology, Allergy and Rheumatology, University of Cincinnati College of Medicine, Cincinnati, Ohio

I. LEONARD BERNSTEIN, MD
Clinical Professor of Medicine and Environmental Health, Division of Immunology, Allergy and Rheumatology, University of Cincinnati College of Medicine, Cincinnati, Ohio

JONATHAN A. BERNSTEIN, MD
Division of Immunology/Allergy Section, Department of Internal Medicine, University of Cincinnati College of Medicine, Cincinnati, Ohio

STUART M. BROOKS, MD
Colleges of Public Health and Medicine, USF Health Science Center, University of South Florida, Tampa, Florida

ANDRÉ CARTIER, MD
Hôpital du Sacré-Cœur de Montréal, Montreal, Quebec, Canada

JORDAN N. FINK, MD
Professor of Pediatrics and Medicine (Allergy/Immunology), Department of Pediatrics, Medical College of Wisconsin, Milwaukee, Wisconsin

ZANA L. LUMMUS, PhD
Adjunct Professor, Department of Internal Medicine, University of Cincinnati College of Medicine, Cincinnati, Ohio

JEAN-LUC MALO, MD
Department of Chest Medicine, Hôpital du Sacré-Cœur, Université de Montréal, Montreal, Quebec, Canada

KARIN A. PACHECO, MD, MSPH
Department of Medicine, National Jewish Health, Denver; Colorado School of Public Health, University of Colorado, Aurora, Colorado

SANTIAGO QUIRCE, MD
Department Allergy, Hospital La Paz Health Research Institute (IdiPAZ), Madrid, Spain

JOAQUIN SASTRE, MD, PhD
Allergy Department, Fundación Jiménez Díaz, Madrid, Spain

ANDREW M. SMITH, MD, MS
Assistant Professor of Clinical Medicine, Department of Internal Medicine, Division of Immunology, University of Cincinnati; Chief of the Allergy Section, Cincinnati Veterans Affairs Medical Center, Cincinnati, Ohio

J. WESLEY SUBLETT, MD, MPH
Division of Immunology, Allergy and Rheumatology, University of Cincinnati College of Medicine, Cincinnati, Ohio

SUSAN M. TARLO, MB BS, FRCP(C)
Department of Medicine, University of Toronto, and Dalla Lana School of Public Health, Toronto Western Hospital, Toronto, Ontario, Canada

OLIVIER VANDENPLAS, MD, PhD
Department of Chest Medicine, Cliniques de Mont-Godinne, Université Catholique de Louvain, Yvoir, Belgium

ADAM V. WISNEWSKI, PhD
Associate Professor, Department of Internal Medicine, Yale School of Medicine, New Haven, Connecticut

MICHAEL C. ZACHARISEN, MD
Professor of Pediatrics and Medicine (Allergy/Immunology), Department of Pediatrics, Medical College of Wisconsin, Milwaukee, Wisconsin

Contents

> The workplace can trigger or induce asthma and cause the onset of different types of work-related asthma (WRA). Based on current knowledge of clinical features, pathophysiologic mechanisms, and evidence supporting a causal relationship, the following conditions should be distinguished in the spectrum of WRA: (1) immunologic occupational asthma (OA), (2) non-immunologic OA, (3) work-exacerbated asthma, and (4) variant syndromes, including eosinophilic bronchitis, potroom asthma, and asthmalike disorders caused by organic dusts. The rationale, issues, and controversies relating to this approach are critically reviewed to stimulate the development of a consensus on operational definitions of the various phenotypes of WRA.

> Much has been learned from epidemiologic studies conducted in the past 4 decades that can be directly applied to the management of workers affected with occupational asthma. Studies have provided information about host factors, environmental exposure, and occupational agents posing the highest risks for development of severe irreversible airway obstruction and asthma disability. Investigators have developed methods for screening workers at risk and novel interventions that may prevent new cases among exposed worker populations. Less is known about the natural history and chronic morbidity associated with work-aggravated asthma and irritant-induced asthma syndromes; more studies are needed in at-risk worker populations.

> International reviews suggest that the median proportion of adult cases of asthma attributable to occupational exposure is between 10% and 15%. Therefore, it is essential that clinicians have a broad knowledge of the various causes associated with occupational asthma. Occupational asthmagens are categorized as low-molecular-weight (LMW, $\leq$1000 kd) and high-molecular-weight (HMW, $\geq$1000 kd) antigens. The purpose of this article is to review the most common representative LMW and HMW causes of occupational asthma over the past 70 years, with specific emphasis on newer causes reported over the past 5 years.

Occupational asthma (OA) is one of the most common forms of work-related lung disease in all industrialized nations. The clinical management of patients with OA depends on an understanding of the multifactorial pathogenetic mechanisms that can contribute to this disease. This article discusses the various immunologic and nonimmunologic mechanisms and genetic susceptibility factors that drive the inflammatory processes of OA.

Occupational asthma (OA) is defined as asthma caused by sources and conditions attributable to a particular occupational environment and not to stimuli encountered outside the workplace. Two types of OA are distinguished based on their appearance after a latency period or not. The most frequent type appears after a latency period leading to sensitization; the clinical assessment of this type of OA is the topic of this review. The differential diagnosis of OA is also reviewed, including work-exacerbated asthma, eosinophilic bronchitis, hyperventilation syndrome, vocal cord dysfunction, bronchiolitis, and other causes of dyspnea or cough.

The management of work-related asthma has some differences from management of other asthma. Components of management include not only making as accurate a diagnosis as possible, identifying the causative agent or triggers at work, and managing the asthma with pharmacologic treatment as for other patients with asthma, but also advising on the appropriate work changes that may be needed, assisting the worker with appropriate compensation claims, and supporting protective measures for coworkers. This article discusses the approaches that may be taken for patients with different forms of work-related asthma.

Thousands of persons experience accidental high-level irritant exposures each year but most recover and few die. Irritants function differently than allergens because their actions proceed nonspecifically and by nonimmunologic mechanisms. For some individuals, the consequence of a single massive exposure to an irritant, gas, vapor or fume is persistent airway hyperresponsiveness and the clinical picture of asthma, referred to as reactive airways dysfunction syndrome (RADS). Repeated irritant exposures may lead to chronic cough and continual airway hyperresponsiveness. Cases of asthma attributed to repeated irritant-exposures may be the result of genetic and/or host factors.

Hypersensitivity pneumonitis can occur from a wide variety of occupational exposures. Although uncommon and difficult to recognize, through a detailed work exposure history, physical examination, radiography, pulmonary function studies, and selected laboratory studies using sera and bronchoalveolar lavage fluid, workers can be identified early to effect avoidance of the antigen and institute pharmacologic therapy, if necessary. A lung biopsy may be necessary to rule out other interstitial lung diseases. Despite the varied organic antigen triggers, the presentation is similar with acute, subacute, or chronic forms. Systemic corticosteroids are the only reliable pharmacologic treatment but do not alter the long-term outcome.

Work-related rhinitis, which includes work-exacerbated rhinitis and occupational rhinoconjunctivitis (OR), is two to three times more common than occupational asthma. High molecular weight proteins and low molecular weight chemicals have been implicated as causes of OR. The diagnosis of work-related rhinitis is established based on occupational history and documentation of immunoglobulin E (IgE) mediated sensitization to the causative agent if possible. Management of work-related rhinitis is similar to that of other causes of rhinitis and includes elimination or reduction of exposure to causative agents combined with pharmacotherapy. If allergens are commercially available, allergen immunotherapy can be considered.

FORTHCOMING ISSUES

RECENT ISSUES

RELATED INTEREST

Infectious Disease Clinics of North America (Volume 25, Issue 2, June 2011)
Global Health, Global Health Education, and Infectious Disease: The New Millennium, Part I
Anvar Velji, MD, *Guest Editor*

THE CLINICS ARE NOW AVAILABLE ONLINE!

Access your subscription at:
www.theclinics.com

Foreword

When the Workplace Air Makes Me Wheeze— Occupational Asthma

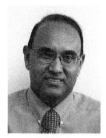

Rafeul Alam, MD, PhD
Consulting Editor

First recognized by Hippocrates, fully described by Bernardino Ramazzini, and scientifically researched by Jack Pepys, occupational asthma remains the most prevalent occupational lung disease despite the implementation of governmental regulatory processes at the workplace. Its incidence remains largely unchanged. This is likely due to the introduction of an increasing number of novel chemicals into the workplace. Occupational asthma distinguishes itself from other forms of asthma in a number of important aspects. There is a well-defined exposure to an offending agent and duration of the exposure. The chemical nature of the offending agent is usually known. Further, the time of onset of asthma is known. These attributes make occupational asthma a highly desirable subject for research.

The induction of asthma by occupational agents with and without a latency period has challenged the classic immunologic dogma of sensitization for many years. Immunological sensitization usually requires a latency period. Another challenge has been the mechanism of T-cell sensitization to small molecular weight compounds. Until recently, we believed that immunological sensitization to non-protein chemicals primarily relied on haptenization of endogenous proteins. This is likely true in some, but not all, cases. Our understanding of immunological sensitization to non-protein chemicals has been undergoing dramatic changes. New immunological paradigms have been established that allow direct recognition of and sensitization to non-protein chemicals such as lipids, glycolipids, and inorganic small molecules.[1,2] These novel paradigms will help us understand the immunological basis of asthma with many occupational agents.

Supported by NIH grants R01AI091614, R56AI077535, PPG HL 36577, and N01 HHSN272200700048C.

Immunol Allergy Clin N Am 31 (2011) ix–x
doi:10.1016/j.iac.2011.08.002
0889-8561/11/$ – see front matter © 2011 Elsevier Inc. All rights reserved.

We have invited leading experts and scholars to update us on the latest in occupational asthma. This effort is led by Dr David Bernstein, an internationally recognized leader in occupational asthma. I hope you will enjoy this issue.

Rafeul Alam, MD, PhD
Division of Allergy and Immunology
National Jewish Health and
University of Colorado Denver Health Sciences Center
1400 Jackson Street
Denver, CO 80206, USA

E-mail address:
AlamR@NJHealth.org

REFERENCES

1. Godfrey DI, Rossjohn J, McCluskey J. The fidelity, occasional promiscuity, and versatility of T cell receptor recognition. Immunity 2008;28:304–14.
2. Chessman D, Kostenko L, Lethborg T, et al. Human leukocyte antigen class I-restricted activation of CD8+ T cells provides the immunogenetic basis of a systemic drug hypersensitivity. Immunity 2008;28(6):822–32.

Preface

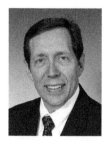

David I. Bernstein, MD
Guest Editor

Work-related asthma is the most common form of occupational lung disease, affecting 10–25% of the adult population. These conditions take on greater importance in industrialized countries but are even more significant in the developing world, which has seen tremendous growth in manufacturing of all kinds. Patients and workers with increased asthma symptoms at work may present to occupational physicians, allergists, or pulmonologists. This monograph, authored by a renowned group of experts, has been written for all physicians with special interests in occupational lung disease, although it is not intended as a comprehensive review. Rather the aim of this issue of *Immunology and Allergy Clinics of North America* is to update selected and timely topics in this field.

Agreement over common definitions for the various work-related asthma syndromes is an essential requisite for evaluating very complicated patients or investigation of these disorders. Drs Malo and Vandenplas introduce this monograph by delineating current definitions work-related asthma and carefully differentiate "work-aggravated asthma" from occupational asthma induced at work. Occupational asthma is very familiar to most clinicians and is now subclassified as: 1) asthma induced by workplace sensitizers; and 2) irritant-induced asthma beginning after acute work-related exposure to high levels of an irritating substance (aka, Reactive Airways Dysfunction Syndrome). New knowledge pertaining to irritant-induced airways disorders is comprehensively addressed by Drs Brooks and Bernstein. In others articles, authoritative authors provide up-to-date reviews of epidemiology, well-recognized and novel etiologic agents, pathogenesis, work-related hypersensitivity pneumonitis, and occupational rhinitis. In their respective articles, Drs Cartier, Sastre, Pacheco, and Tarlo provide practical and rational approaches for the clinician consultant on the clinical assessment and management of work-related asthma.

I would like to acknowledge and thank the esteemed group of authors represented in this monograph for their contributions. Finally, we must recognize the small cadre of researchers all over the globe whose scientific contributions during the past 50 years

Immunol Allergy Clin N Am 31 (2011) xi–xii
doi:10.1016/j.iac.2011.08.001
0889-8561/11/$ – see front matter © 2011 Elsevier Inc. All rights reserved.

immunology.theclinics.com

continue to build our knowledge of occupational lung disorders and improve the health of workers at risk.

David I. Bernstein, MD
Division of Immunology, Allergy and Rheumatology
University of Cincinnati College of Medicine
3255 Eden Avenue
Cincinnati, OH 45267-0563, USA

E-mail address:
bernstdd@ucmail.uc.edu

Definitions and Classification of Work-Related Asthma

Jean-Luc Malo, MD[a],*, Olivier Vandenplas, MD, PhD[b]

KEYWORDS

- Asthma • Bronchial hyperresponsiveness
- Occupational disease • Irritant-induced asthma
- Reactive airways dysfunction syndrome

The expression occupational asthma (OA) was originally the only term used to describe the link, most often causal, between asthma and the workplace. Moreover, OA then included only the form that occurred after a latency period and the onset of sensitization. However, in recent years, a more general approach that encompasses all conditions that link asthma to the workplace, not only having a causal relationship but also playing a role in asthma exacerbations, has been proposed and is being labeled work-related asthma (WRA) (**Fig. 1**). Another type of OA has also been recognized, the type caused by inhalational accidents and causing acute irritation of the airways. Variants have also been described, especially occupational eosinophilic bronchitis. In the same way as the existence of a consensus definition of asthma[1] has improved its recognition and management, precise and workable definitions of OA and other types of WRA are required to improve the investigation and management of these conditions.

This article is an update of a previously published article[2] that aims at delineating the different phenotypes of WRA based on currently available evidence.

NOSOLOGIC DEFINITIONS OF WRA

There is now a wide consensus that WRA should be disentangled into several well-characterized and less-well-characterized phenotypes.[3,4] Considering that the keystone for defining OA is the causal relationship between workplace exposure and the

Funding: OV is supported by a grant from the Actions de recherche concertées de la Communauté française de Belgique.

[a] Department of Chest Medicine, Hôpital du Sacré-Cœur, Université de Montréal, 5400 West Gouin Boulevard, Montreal H4J 1C5, Canada

[b] Department of Chest Medicine, Cliniques de Mont-Godinne, Université Catholique de Louvain, 1 Avenue G. Therasse, B5530 Yvoir, Belgium

* Corresponding author.

E-mail address: malojl@meddir.umontreal.ca

doi:10.1016/j.iac.2011.07.003
immunology.theclinics.com

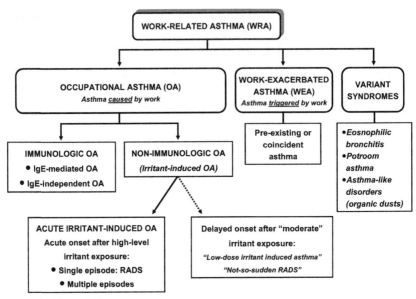

Fig. 1. Definition of WRA.

development of asthma[5–12] as summarized in **Table 1**, the term OA should be restricted to those conditions inducing asthma or caused by the person's occupation.

OA

OA is a disease characterized by airway inflammation, variable airflow limitation, and airway hyperresponsiveness caused by conditions attributable to a particular occupational environment and not to stimuli encountered outside the workplace.[3] This type of WRA would be more appropriately labeled occupation-induced asthma to emphasize the determining causal relationship between asthma and the workplace. Two types of OA can be distinguished depending on whether they seem to be mediated by immunologic mechanisms or not: immunologic OA and nonimmunologic OA.

Immunologic OA

Immunologic OA is characterized by WRA appearing after a latency period of exposure necessary to acquire immunologically mediated sensitization to the causal agent. This category encompasses (1) OA caused by all high-molecular-weight (HMW) and certain low-molecular-weight (LMW) agents (eg, platinum salts, acid anhydrides, reactive dyes, sulfonechloramide, and obeche wood) for which an immunologic (IgE mediated) mechanism has been proven, and (2) OA induced by LMW occupational agents, such as diisocyanates, Western red cedar, or acrylates, acting through largely uncertain immunologic mechanisms. This entity has also been termed sensitizer-induced OA in the recent guidelines issued by the American College of Chest Physicians.[4] According to the nomenclature proposed by the European Academy of Allergy and Clinical Immunology,[13] OA mediated by immunologic mechanisms (whatever their precise nature) that results in clinical allergic hypersensitivity should be termed allergic OA. When there is evidence of IgE-mediated mechanisms, the term should be IgE-mediated allergic OA.

Table 1
Comparison of historical definitions of OA

Study	Definition of Asthma	Nature of the Relationship Between Asthma and Work	Causal Agents	Mechanisms
Pepys,[5] 1980	"Widespread reversible airway obstruction"	"Widespread reversible airway obstruction" (?)	not mentioned	not mentioned
Newman-Taylor,[6] 1980	"Variable airways narrowing"	"causally related to"	"airborne dust, gases, vapors, or fumes"	"clinical criteria of hypersensitivity"
Parkes,[7] 1982	not mentioned	"caused by"	"specific agent in the form of dust, fumes, or vapors"	not mentioned
Brooks,[8] 1985	"Generalized obstruction of the airways, usually reversible"	"caused by"	"substance or material that a worker manufactures or uses directly or is incidentally present at the workplace"	not mentioned
Cotes and Steel,[9] 1987	not mentioned	"caused by"	"sensitizing bronchoconstrictor substance"	sensitization
Chan-Yeung and Malo,[10] 1987	"Asthma"	"caused by"	"specific agents in the workplace"	"exclusion of bronchoconstriction induced by irritants at work"
Burge,[11] 1988	"Asthma"	"due, in whole or in part to"	"agents met at work"	"sensitization"
Chan-Yeung,[99] ACCP consensus statement, 1995	"Variable airflow limitation and/or airway hyperresponsiveness"	"due to"	"causes and conditions attributable to a particular occupational environment and not to stimuli encountered outside the workplace"	Immunologic and nonimmunologic
American Thoracic Society Statement,[64] 2004	"Asthma"	"caused by"	"Work exposure"	Sensitization, RADS, and nonimmunologic airway irritation in subjects with preexisting asthma (ie, irritant-induced asthma)
Bernstein et al,[3] 2006	"Variable airflow limitation and/or airway hyperresponsiveness and/or airway inflammation"	"due to"	"causes and conditions attributable to a particular occupational environment and not to stimuli encountered outside the workplace"	Immunologic and nonimmunologic

Nonimmunologic OA

Nonimmunologic OA is characterized by the absence of a latency period needed for the acquisition of sensitization as in immunologic OA because asthma develops within hours after a single exposure to inhaled irritants at very high concentrations at the workplace. This clinical entity was initially described under the label reactive airways dysfunction syndrome (RADS), and, subsequently, the term irritant-induced asthma was introduced to denote asthma occurring after a single or multiple high-level exposures to irritants.[14] The diagnosis of RADS requires all the following criteria[15]: (1) identification of date, times, frequency, and extent of exposure; (2) onset of symptoms within 24 hours of exposure; (3) no latency period; (4) symptoms less likely to improve away from work; and (5) presence of airflow obstruction and/or presence and persistence of nonspecific bronchial hyperresponsiveness (NSBH). Such nonimmunologic types of asthma that are causally related to the workplace should be labeled nonallergic OA.

Work-exacerbated Asthma

Work-exacerbated asthma (WEA), also termed work-aggravated asthma, is preexisting or concurrent asthma that is exacerbated by workplace exposure. As proposed, the term WEA refers to asthma triggered by various work-related factors (eg, common aeroallergens, irritants, or exercise) in workers who are known to have preexisting or concurrent asthma (ie, asthma that is occurring at the same time but is not caused by workplace exposures).[4] Workers with WEA (1) report worsening of their asthmatic symptoms at work and improvement away from work, (2) are often exposed to chemicals at work, (3) more often use their rescue bronchodilator at work, (4) may show an increased neutrophilic inflammation while at work (by comparison with OA in which eosinophilic inflammation is more often found), and (5) suffer from the same adverse socioeconomic consequences as workers with OA.[16,17]

Variant Syndromes

Occupational eosinophilic bronchitis

Eosinophilic bronchitis has been increasingly described as a cause of chronic cough, which is characterized by sputum eosinophilia (>3% of nonsquamous cells), but, unlike asthma, evidence of variable airflow obstruction and/or NSBH is lacking.[18] Eosinophilic bronchitis has been causally related to several occupational agents, such as latex, wheat flour, α-amylase, egg lysozyme, isocyanates, acrylates, formaldehyde, chloramine-T, epoxy resin hardener, stainless steel welding fumes, and mushroom spores.[19] The mechanisms leading to the absence of NSBH despite the eosinophilic bronchial inflammation remain uncertain.[20–22] The natural history of work-related eosinophilic bronchitis is unknown, and it should be determined whether this syndrome can progress to typical OA.[23,24] Eosinophilic bronchitis should be considered as an occupationally induced condition when the work-related changes in sputum eosinophils are significant and reproducible.

Potroom asthma

The term potroom asthma refers to the occurrence of WRA symptoms among those employed in the production of aluminum from alumina into electrolytic cells (pots).[25] Potroom asthma develops after a symptom-free period (latency), and asthma symptoms usually occur several hours after work exposure and improve away from work. However, potroom asthma is not included in OA because different mechanisms could be involved in the development of this entity, including an irritant effect resulting from exposure to pollutants (ie, hydrogen fluoride, sulfur dioxide) and an immunologically mediated reaction directed against trace amounts of metals. Work-related changes in peak expiratory flow have been described in symptomatic potroom workers, although most of these workers failed to demonstrate significant NSBH during workplace exposure. Only one report documented the development of a biphasic asthmatic reaction associated with an increase in NSBH on exposure to the potroom environment.[26] Bronchial biopsy results of subjects with potroom asthma revealed the presence of airway inflammation and airway remodeling similar to what has been described in other types of asthma.[27]

Asthmalike disorders

Exposure to vegetable dusts (grain, cotton, and other textile fibers) and dust from animal confinement buildings can induce asthmalike and systemic symptoms associated with acute decrement in expiratory flows, transient increase in NSBH, and neutrophilic airway inflammation.[28,29] These endotoxin-related conditions share common features that differentiate them from OA: (1) there are systemic symptoms that are not generally present in OA, (2) there is no latency period and symptoms can occur in naive subjects on first exposure, (3) the severity of the symptoms typically decreases over the working week (tolerance), (4) cross-shift changes in expiratory flows are less pronounced, (5) NSBH is neither a prominent nor a persistent feature, and (6) these conditions are associated with a predominant neutrophilic airway inflammation.

RATIONALE FOR DEFINING DIFFERENT PHENOTYPES OF WRA

WRA is the broad term that refers to asthma that is exacerbated or induced by inhalation exposures in the workplace.[4] Within this broad spectrum of asthma conditions related to the workplace, several entities can be identified based on the strength of the causal relationship, clinical features, and/or pathophysiologic mechanisms (**Table 2**).

Causal Relationship Between Asthma and Work

All previously published definitions of OA (see **Table 1**)[5–12] stipulate that there should be a causal relationship between workplace exposure and asthma and that the causal agent (identified or not) should be specific to the workplace. A causal relationship between workplace exposure and asthma implies that agents causing OA should be able to induce the development of the characteristic features of asthma, including variable airflow limitation, NSBH, and airway inflammation.[1] However, advances in the pathophysiologic mechanisms of asthma have clearly indicated the various outcomes for agents that cause airway inflammation and NSBH, described as inducers, and for those that trigger airway narrowing in subjects with NSBH, without inducing airway inflammation, labeled inciters.[30] Conceptually, only inducers can be considered to be causal agents because they induce not only airflow obstruction but also changes in airway inflammation and NSBH, whereas inciters increase the frequency of asthma symptoms in those with preexisting or coincidental asthma. The prototypes of asthma inducers are common aeroallergens acting through an IgE-mediated mechanism. Acute exposure to these agents in the laboratory can provoke immediate and/or late asthmatic reactions and, although not invariably so, an increase in NSBH and airway inflammation.[31,32] Furthermore, exposure to inducers at doses that do not elicit airflow obstruction can provoke an increase in NSBH and airway inflammation, which can be assumed to result in a worsening of the asthma condition.[33,34]

Establishing the causal relationship between asthma and the workplace should therefore take into account the distinction between inciters and inducers. Numerous agents present in the workplace can be considered to be asthma inducers because

Table 2
Nosologic categorization of WRA

Criteria	OA		Irritant-Induced Asthma	WEA	Variant Syndromes
	Immunologic OA	Nonimmunologic OA (Acute Irritant-Induced Asthma)			EB, ALD, PA,
Mechanisms	IgE-mediated: HMW and some LMW agents; uncertain: most LMW agents	Acute toxic injury from single (RADS) or multiple high-level irritant exposures	Unknown	Unknown	EB, immunologic; ALD, endotoxins; PA, unknown
Clinical features	Latency period, clinical criteria for hypersensitivity to a specific occupational agent	Sudden onset, no latency period (RADS), no work-related symptoms[a]	No work-related symptoms	WRA symptoms (preexisting or coincident asthma)[b]	EB, work-related cough; ALD, systemic symptoms; PA, work-related respiratory symptoms
Evidence of a causal relationship	Empirical ascertainment in individuals (inhalation challenges)	Inference from temporal relationship between acute exposures and onset of asthma	Epidemiologic association between work and an excess risk of asthma (ie, work-attributable asthma), eg, cleaning asthma	Lack of objective test, exclusion of immunologic OA	EB, work-related sputum eosinophilia; ALD, work-related changes in FEV1; PA, none

Abbreviations: ALD, asthmalike disorders induced by vegetable dusts (cotton, textile fibers, grain); EB, eosinophilic bronchitis; FEV1, forced expiratory volume in 1 second; PA, potroom asthma.
[a] With the possibility of subjects who develop WEA after the inception of RADS.
[b] Subjects with immunologic or nonimmunologic OA may subsequently develop WEA.

they have been documented as causing asthmatic reactions, airway inflammation, and NSBH.[35] These agents encompass a wide variety of HMW protein allergens as well as LMW substances. In subjects with OA, exposure to these agents can cause an increase in NSBH and airway inflammation, even in the absence of airway obstruction.[36,37]

In recent years, studies have confirmed that exposure to very high concentrations of irritant materials can also lead to the development of NSBH and airway inflammation and cause what has been labeled RADS by Brooks and coworkers.[38] RADS shares many features with asthma because of a sensitizing mechanism. In this specific case, the causal relationship can often be ascertained by the clinical history: exposure to high concentrations of an agent causes respiratory symptoms, cough being common, in the minutes or hours after the inhalational accident. After several years, the symptoms and functional changes (ie, airway obstruction and NSBH) are comparable to what is found in asthma.[39] Furthermore, bronchial biopsy results show inflammatory and structural features similar to common asthma.[40] By contrast, exposure of subjects with asthma to lower concentrations of irritants does not generally induce changes in NSBH or airway inflammation,[41–43] with the noticeable exception of ozone.[44]

Categorizing various forms of asthma related to work exposure according to the strength of their causal relationship with the workplace environment is relevant not only for scientific reasons but also for medical, preventive, and medicolegal purposes. Asthma caused by inducers that act through a sensitizing process generally requires complete removal from workplace exposure because persistence of exposure to these agents can result in the progressive worsening of the characteristic features of asthma and long-term functional impairment.[45] However, such therapeutic and preventive options are associated with significant professional, financial, and social consequences.[46]

Pathophysiologic Mechanisms

A wide variety of occupational agents have been identified as causing a form of asthma that meets the clinical criteria for hypersensitivity: (1) WRA symptoms develop only after an initial symptom-free period of exposure, (2) asthmatic reactions tend to recur on reexposure to the causal agent at concentrations not affecting others similarly exposed, and (3) asthma affects only a proportion (usually a minority) of those exposed to the agent.[6] Accordingly, some definitions of OA have specified that the agent causing OA should exert its effects through sensitization.[9,11] The use of the term sensitization may suggest that the immunologic mechanism has been precisely characterized. However, the mechanisms leading to the development of OA caused by most LMW substances remain largely unknown,[47] although there is evidence that immunologic processes mediated by T lymphocytes could be involved independently from the production of specific IgE antibodies.

Although immunologic mechanisms may well be involved in the development of RADS, as suggested by less-important inflammation induced by chlorine exposure in γ T cell–deficient mice by comparison with wild mice,[48] the original insult is purely an acute toxic injury of the airways. Although the functional and pathologic features of immunologically mediated OA are indistinguishable from those of common asthma, whether allergic or nonallergic, the features of RADS show some differences. The presence of a latency period (ie, a period of exposure necessary to acquire immunologic sensitization) has been proposed as a key feature to differentiate immunologic OA characterized clinically by bronchial hyperresponsiveness to occupational agents from asthma caused by acute exposure to high concentrations of irritants (RADS), irrespective of the underlying pathophysiologic mechanisms.[12] After the initial event, the reversibility of airway obstruction is not as constant or as marked in subjects with RADS as in those with OA or nonoccupational asthma.[49] However, the natural history seems similar to that of immunologic OA, with an apparent cure in approximately 25% of subjects assessed 2 years or more after the inhalational accident.[39,50] Although the chronic pathologic features show eosinophilic infiltration as for asthma, there is more airway remodeling than in standard asthma.[40]

ISSUES AND CONTROVERSIES
Immunologic OA

The causal role of occupational agents in the development of immunologic OA can be experimentally/empirically documented in an individual case by demonstrating, through inhalation challenges in the laboratory or at the workplace, that exposure to a specific agent induces the characteristic features of asthma (ie, airway obstruction, NSBH, and airway inflammation). Showing that this agent does not elicit such effects in other subjects with asthma provides further evidence that the agent is an inducer rather than an inciter of asthma. There are, however, several discussion issues related to documenting the causal relationship between a workplace agent and asthma.

Preexisting asthma

Although this is not common, immunologic OA can undoubtedly develop in workers whose asthma preexisted to the workplace exposure, leading to the possibility of OA superimposed on previous nonoccupational asthma. Noticeably, the presence of NSBH before employment is associated with an increased risk for the development of OA caused by some HMW agents.[51] Therefore, a history of asthma (allergic or nonallergic, quiescent or symptomatic) before entering the incriminated workplace cannot be used to discriminate between immunologic OA and WEA. Prospective cohort studies have demonstrated that agents causing immunologic OA can induce asthma de novo.[51,52] However, on an individual basis, unless a worker has been prospectively assessed in a surveillance program, it cannot be formally proven that the occupational environment caused asthma de novo after entering a particular workplace. The inception of the characteristic features of asthma can be demonstrated only a posteriori by showing the resurgence of NSBH after inhalation challenges with the causal agent in subjects with OA in whom NSBH has returned to a normal level after removal from exposure.[53]

Characteristic features of asthma

Determining which of the characteristic features of asthma (ie, variable airway obstruction, NSBH, and airway inflammation) should be required for establishing causality in clinical practice remains a difficult issue. The occurrence of late or dual asthmatic reactions after exposure to an occupational agent strongly supports an immunologic mechanism, but it may be difficult to differentiate immediate bronchial responses provoked by inducers from those triggered by irritant substances, although the responses provoked by irritant substances are usually less reproducible and resolve faster than those provoked by inducers. A postchallenge increase in NSBH provides further evidence for immunologic OA, although this is not a consistent finding.[31] Furthermore, it has been increasingly acknowledged that subjects with OA may fail to exhibit NSBH both before and after asthmatic reactions induced by occupational agents.[53–56] This absence of NSBH in a worker with OA as confirmed by specific challenges is generally because it is assessed at a time when the worker is no longer at work. In some workers, enhanced NSBH can be brief and disappear in the hours after cessation of exposure at work or at the time of specific inhalation challenges. The induction of an eosinophilic airway inflammation can be considered a specific marker of airway responses mediated by immunologic mechanisms.[19] Most asthmatic reactions elicited by occupational agents acting through an immunologic mechanism are associated with an increase in sputum eosinophils, which may even precede the changes in airway caliber and NSBH.[19,56] However, analysis of induced sputum is not widely available, and approximately 20% of subjects cannot produce interpretable sputum. Measurement of exhaled nitric oxide as a surrogate of eosinophilic inflammation is much less sensitive.[57] An increase in sputum neutrophil counts has been reported in subjects with OA due to LMW agents, especially diisocyanates.[58,59] A neutrophilic airway inflammation is not specific for immunologic OA because it has been described after exposure to irritant compounds such as ozone,[60] diesel exhaust particles,[61] and endotoxin.[62,63]

Agents specific to the workplace

Some published definitions of WRA stated that agents causing OA should be specific to the workplace.[4,10,12,64–69] However, common inhalant allergens may also be present in high concentrations in occupational environments (eg, molds in building renovation or waste processing workers, pets in animal care workers, and house dust mites in domestic cleaners). These allergens can induce a worsening of asthma in subjects with previously documented sensitization, which should be regarded as either WEA, because the agent is ubiquitous and not specific to the workplace, or even OA, because the mechanism is clearly immunologic. On the other hand, it is not possible to demonstrate or rule out that workplace exposure to common allergens has contributed to the initiation of immunologic OA in subjects without preexisting asthma or atopic status.

Nonimmunologic OA

It is now widely accepted that exposure to very high levels of an irritant gas, fume, aerosol, or vapor at work can induce the development of asthma.[4,10,12,64–69] Recent guidelines[4,64,65] and review articles[12,66–69] have acknowledged that the most definitive form of asthma induced by respiratory irritants is RADS, which refers to the acute onset of asthma after a single high-level irritant exposure.[38] Although widely used, the term RADS is not indicative of the nature and mechanisms of the disorder, which suggests that it should be replaced by acute irritant-induced asthma[70] to avoid further confusion with delayed or progressive forms of asthma associated with irritant exposures at work. In the case of acute irritant-induced OA, the causal role of the workplace can be ascertained by the strong temporal association between an inhalation accident and the rapid onset of asthma. By contrast, there is still controversy about the characteristics and work-relatedness of other forms of the so-called irritant-induced asthma.

Accidental aggravation of asthma

According to the criteria initially proposed by Brooks and colleagues[38] and recently adapted by the American College of Chest Physicians guidelines,[4] a diagnosis of RADS cannot be made in subjects with preexisting asthma. It is, nevertheless, conceivable that high-level exposure to irritants can induce similar adverse effects in asthmatic and healthy subjects. Therefore, the reactivation of asthma in remission or the persistent worsening of preexisting stable asthma should be considered as possible consequences of an acute inhalation injury at work.[71–73] There is some suggestion from the Ontario Workers' Compensation Board that worsening of preexisting asthma induced by high-level inhalation of irritants, termed accidental aggravation of asthma by the investigators,[73] may have different clinical characteristics compared with RADS. Whether accidental aggravation of asthma should be categorized as acute irritant-induced OA or as a particular phenotype of WEA remains debatable.

Repeated high-level exposures

Clinical series have suggested that the development of asthma can result from multiple exposures rather than a single exposure to high levels of irritants.[14,74,75] Some of the subjects described in these series had WRA symptoms and/or work-related changes in NSBH or in expiratory peak flow values, suggesting a possible misclassification of immunologic OA or WEA.[14,75] In addition, analysis of reported subjects in whom asthma developed after multiple high-level exposures to irritants shows that the initiation of asthma actually resulted from a single high-level exposure requiring emergency room treatment, which is consistent with classic RADS.[74] Surveys of workers repeatedly exposed to high levels of chlorine,[76,77] ozone,[78] and sulfur dioxide[79] found that severe symptomatic gassing episodes were associated with an increased incidence of NSBH or adult-onset asthma. In the European Community Respiratory Health Survey, inhalation accidents, such as fire, mixing cleaning products, or chemical spills, were associated with a 3.3-fold increased risk of new-onset asthma.[80] Accordingly, asthma resulting from multiple high-level exposures to irritant substances can be categorized as nonimmunologic OA, provided that the onset of persistent asthma symptoms can be temporally related to 1 documented severe inhalation accident. Noteworthy in such conditions of multiple exposures to irritants is that the absence of a latency period should no longer be regarded as a key clinical feature for distinguishing nonimmunologic from immunologic OA.

Irritant-induced asthma

Tarlo and Broder[14] introduced the term irritant-induced asthma to characterize workers who develop asthma after both single and multiple high-level irritant exposures. The guidelines for assessing and managing asthma risk at work, at school, and during recreation issued by the American Thoracic Society used the term irritant-induced asthma to describe nonimmunologic airway irritation in subjects with preexisting asthma, which can be triggered by a variety of irritating aerosols, dusts, gases and fumes (eg, cleaning materials, chlorine, sulfur dioxide), and exercise.[64] More recently, all cases of new-onset asthma in workers exposed to irritant substances that do not meet the stringent criteria for RADS have been subsumed under the general category of irritant-induced asthma.[4] Such cases may involve individuals in whom asthma had a delayed onset after repeated exposures to moderate or excessive, although poorly documented, concentrations of irritant compounds in the workplace.[81,82] Evidence supporting the work-relatedness of such low-dose irritant asthma or not-so-sudden RADS is still very weak. Case reports are open to clinical biases because they assume that the factor of interest was the cause of the disease in the absence of control data. Epidemiologic studies of workers exposed to irritants (eg, chlorine, ozone, and sulfur dioxide) documented a role of acute symptomatic gassing accidents in the development of asthma but not of moderate-level exposures to irritants.[76–79] Accordingly, the constellation of poorly characterized asthma syndromes that are currently classified under the ambiguous term irritant-induced asthma cannot be considered as OA because the causal relationship between workplace exposure and the development of asthma is not supported by available scientific evidence, and this relationship cannot be ascertained with a sufficient level of confidence on an individual basis.

WEA

The term WEA is widely used to denote the worsening of preexisting or coincident (new onset) asthma as a result of workplace environmental exposure.[3,4,65,66,69,83] WEA is now widely accepted as a form of asthma related to the workplace (WRA) but not caused by the workplace.

WEA is characterized by an increase in the frequency or severity of self-reported asthma symptoms and/or an increase in medication use temporally related to work exposure. More severe exacerbations may lead to increased health care visits. These clinical features are similar to those of immunologic OA, which may lead to misclassification of OA as WEA when appropriate investigations are not performed. Thus, a substantial proportion of subjects who experience exacerbation of asthma symptoms at work fail to demonstrate objective evidence of asthma worsening when they are exposed to their workplace or to the suspected agent in the laboratory.[84–86] A limited number of studies have examined the clinical characteristics of patients with WEA. From clinical series in which specific inhalation challenge was used to separate WEA from OA, investigators found quite similar indices of disease severity for both conditions.[87–89]

Conceptually, a worsening of asthma at work could be documented by objective physiologic changes related to work. In one study, researchers observed that about half of WEA cases had serial peak expiratory flow measurements that were more variable while working compared with periods away from work, although these measurements were not able to differentiate WEA from OA.[89] In addition, assessments of lung function tests to support the work relatedness of asthma are much less frequently conducted for WEA cases (11%) than for OA cases (76%), as suggested by a review of WRA cases in the Canadian province of Ontario.[90] It should be noted, however, that OA and WEA are not mutually exclusive, meaning that someone with OA can subsequently experience WEA. One study suggested that WEA seems to be characterized by an increase in sputum neutrophils more than in eosinophils, which is more a feature of OA.[91]

A Task Force of the American Thoracic Society (document in preparation) has recently reviewed the available information pertaining to WEA and proposed a consensus case definition based on the following 4 criteria:

- Criterion 1: preexisting or concurrent asthma. Preexisting asthma is asthma with onset before entering the worksite of interest. Concurrent asthma or coincident asthma is asthma with onset while employed in the worksite of interest but not because of exposures in that worksite.
- Criterion 2: asthma-work temporal relationship. It is necessary to document that the exacerbation of asthma was temporally associated with work, based either on self-reports of symptoms or medication use relative to work or on more objective indicators such as work-related patterns of serial peak expiratory flow rates.
- Criterion 3: conditions exist at work that can exacerbate asthma.
- Criterion 4: asthma caused by work (ie, OA) is unlikely.

Epidemiologic studies conducted in general populations indicate that WEA is a highly prevalent condition, with a median prevalence estimate of 21.5% among adult asthmatics. A wide variety of conditions at work can exacerbate asthma symptoms, including irritant chemicals, dusts, second-hand smoke, common allergens that may be present at work, as well as other exposures, such as emotional stress, worksite temperature, and physical exertion. However, there is a dearth of quantitative exposure data and information about what exposure levels at work can induce worsening of asthma. The pathophysiologic mechanisms leading to WEA remain largely unknown and are probably multiple (eg, neurogenic inflammation triggered by airway epithelium injury, heightened airway sensitivity to chemical and physical stimuli). Noneosinophilic inflammation of the airways might also be involved in the development of WEA because some subjects with this condition show an increase in sputum neutrophils after exposure to the suspected agents at work[91] or in the laboratory.[92]

There is accumulating evidence that the socioeconomic impact of WEA is similar to that resulting from OA in terms of unemployment and loss of labor-derived income.[17,93] In addition, WEA is associated with a higher rate of job changes, a lower quality of life, and a greater use of health care resources compared with asthma unrelated to work.[93] Nevertheless, WEA should be distinguished from OA because the pathophysiologic consequences of these 2 conditions as well as their management approaches differ substantially. Reducing workplace exposure to respiratory irritants and optimizing antiasthma treatment should a priori allow workers with WEA to continue working in the same job while minimizing the adverse socioeconomic impacts. Several challenge studies have shown that changes in airflow limitation induced by exposure (eg, to sulfur dioxide, endotoxin and physical factors) can be reduced or prevented by inhaled bronchodilators, suggesting a possible management component for individuals with asthma in these environments (American Thoracic Society document, in preparation). However, there is still little information on the natural history of WEA and the long-term effects of treatment interventions. Two studies have explored the long-term outcome of WEA cases after cessation of exposure compared with OA.[88,93] Those with WEA and OA showed significant and equivalent improvements in symptom scores and medical resource use, but subjects with WEA showed a trend toward less improvement in NSBH and smaller reduction in the dose of inhaled corticosteroids compared with patients with OA. Subjects with WEA tended to show a decrease in sputum neutrophil counts, whereas those with OA had a trend toward a decrease in sputum eosinophils.

PRACTICAL APPLICATIONS OF THE DEFINITIONS

Recent surveys have consistently found that subjects with WRA remain inappropriately evaluated in both general and specialized medical practices.[90,94,95] These findings emphasize the need for developing working definitions for the various phenotypes of WRA.[70] These definitions can be adapted for different purposes, including clinical evaluation, medicolegal assessment, epidemiologic identification, and workplace surveillance programs. For instance, establishing a clinical diagnosis of OA requires the highest level of evidence because it is associated with considerable medical and socioeconomic consequences.[96] The requirements for identifying OA in workplace surveillance programs and epidemiologic investigation are less stringent than for medical evaluation.

The National Institute for Occupational Safety and Health has developed a surveillance case definition of OA (**Box 1**).[97] However, several limitations of this definition should be considered. The association between documented (new onset) asthma, work-related symptoms, and workplace exposure to agents known to cause asthma (criteria A+B+C3 in **Box 1**) provides only a low predictive value for the presence of OA.[84] The preexisting asthma criterion (criterion C1 in **Box 1**) for defining WEA may result in misdiagnosis of true immunologic OA occurring in subjects with preexisting asthma.

The case definitions[97,98] and diagnostic algorithms for OA[4,99] that have been proposed to date have not formally incorporated the predictive value of the various diagnostic procedures. The authors propose a clinical case definition based on the posttest probability of OA derived from the systematic review conducted by the

---

Box 1
Surveillance case definition of OA proposed by the Sentinel Event Notification Systems for Occupational Risks

A. Health care professional's diagnosis of asthma

B. An association between symptoms of asthma and work

C. One or more of the following criteria

1. Increased asthma symptoms or increased use of asthma medication (on entering an occupational exposure setting) experienced by a person with preexisting asthma who was symptomatic or treated with asthma medication within the 2 years before entering that new occupational setting (work-aggravated asthma)

2. New asthma symptoms that develop within 24 hours after a 1-time high-level inhalation exposure (at work) to an irritant gas, fume, smoke, or vapor and that persist for at least 3 months (RADS)

3. Workplace exposure to an agent or process previously associated with OA

4. Work-related changes in serially measured forced expiratory volume in 1 second or peak expiratory flow rate

5. Work-related changes in bronchial responsiveness as measured by serial nonspecific inhalation challenge testing

6. Positive response to specific inhalation challenge testing with an agent to which the patient has been exposed at work

Data from Jajosky RA, Harrison R, Reinisch F, et al. Surveillance of work-related asthma in selected US states using surveillance guidelines for state health departments—California, Massachusetts, Michigan and New Jersey. MMWR CDC Surveill Summ 1999;48(SS-3):1–20.

Agency for Health care Research and Quality,[100] which provides estimates of the sensitivity and specificity of diagnostic procedures compared with those of specific inhalation challenges.[100]

SUMMARY

The clinical and medicolegal definition of OA should be limited to include only those cases in which a causal relationship can be objectively established between exposure to a workplace or a substance in the workplace and the inception of asthma. This relationship can be established with a sufficient level of evidence for immunologically mediated OA, either through IgE-dependent or IgE-independent mechanisms, and acute irritant-induced OA, the best characterized form of nonimmunologic OA. Other types of asthma related to the workplace environment, including low-dose irritant-induced asthma and WEA, require further investigation to identify their characteristics and to develop evidence-based working definitions.

ACKNOWLEDGMENTS

The authors would like to express their thanks to Kathe Lieber for reviewing the manuscript.

REFERENCES

1. National Heart Lung, and Blood Institute, National Institutes of Health, Bethesda, Maryland 20892. International consensus report on diagnosis and treatment of asthma. Eur Respir J 1992;5:601–41.

2. Vandenplas O, Malo JL. Definitions and types of work-related asthma: a nosological approach. Eur Respir J 2003;21:706–12.

3. Bernstein IL, Chan-Yeung M, Malo JL, et al. Definition and classification of asthma in the workplace. In: Bernstein IL, Chan-Yeung M, Malo JL, et al, editors. Asthma in the workplace. 3rd edition. New York: Taylor & Francis; 2006. p. 1–8.

4. Tarlo SM, Balmes J, Balkisssoon R, et al. ACCP consensus statement: diagnosis and management of work-related asthma. Chest 2008;134:1S–41S.

5. Pepys J. Occupational asthma: review of present clinical and immunologic status. J Allergy Clin Immunol 1980;66:179–85.

6. Newman-Taylor AJ. Occupational asthma. Thorax 1980;35:241–5.

7. Parkes WR. Occupational asthma (including byssinosis). In: Occupational lung disorders. London: Butterworths; 1982. p. 415–53.

8. Brooks SM. Occupational asthma. Chest 1985;87:218S–22S.

9. Cotes JE, Steel J. Occupational asthma. In: Work-related lung disorders. Oxford (United Kingdom): Blackwell Scientific Publications; 1987. p. 345–72.

10. Chan-Yeung M, Malo JL. Occupational asthma. Chest 1987;91:130S–6S.

11. Burge PS. Occupational asthma. In: Barnes P, Rodger IW, Thomson NC, editors. Asthma: basic mechanisms and clinical management. London: Academic Press; 1988. p. 465–82.

12. Bernstein IL, Bernstein DI, Chan-Yeung M, et al. Asthma in the workplace. 3rd edition. New York: Taylor & Francis; 2006.

13. Johansson SG, Hourihane JO, Bousquet J, et al. A revised nomenclature for allergy: an EAACI position statement from the EAACI nomenclature task force. Allergy 2001;56:813–24.

14. Tarlo SM, Broder I. Irritant-induced occupational asthma. Chest 1989;96(2): 297–300.

15. Gautrin D, Bernstein IL, Brooks SM, et al. Reactive airways dysfunction syndrome and irritant-induced asthma. In: Bernstein IL, Chan-Yeung M, Malo JL, et al, editors. Asthma in the workplace. 3rd edition. New York: Taylor & Francis; 2006. p. 579–627.

16. Wagner GR, Henneberger PK. Asthma exacerbated at work. In: Bernstein IL, Chan-Yeung M, Malo JL, et al, editors. Asthma in the workplace. 3rd edition. New York: Taylor & Francis; 2006. p. 631–40.

17. Vandenplas O, Henneberger PK. Socioeconomic outcomes in work-exacerbated asthma. Curr Opin Allergy Clin Immunol 2007;7:236–41.

18. Brightling CE. Chronic cough due to nonasthmatic eosinophilic bronchitis: ACCP evidence-based clinical practice guidelines. Chest 2006;129(Suppl):116S–21S.

19. Quirce S, Lemière C, deBlay F, et al. Noninvasive methods for assessment of airway inflammation in occupational settings. Allergy 2010;65:445–58.

20. Brightling CE, Symon FA, Birring SS, et al. Comparison of airway immunopathology of eosinophilic bronchitis and asthma. Thorax 2003;58:528–32.

21. Berry MA, Parker D, Neale N, et al. Sputum and bronchial submucosal IL-13 expression in asthma and eosinophilic bronchitis. J Allergy Clin Immunol 2004;114:1106–9.

22. Sastre B, Fernández-Nieto M, Mollá R, et al. Increased prostaglandin E2 levels in the airway of patients with eosinophilic bronchitis. Allergy 2008;63:58–66.

23. Park SW, Lee YM, Jang AS, et al. Development of chronic airway obstruction in patients with eosinophilic bronchitis: a prospective follow-up study. Chest 2004; 125:1998–2004.

24. Berry MA, Hargadon B, McKenna S, et al. Observational study of the natural history of eosinophilic bronchitis. Clin Exp Allergy 2005;35:598–601.

25. Kongerud J, Boe J, Soyseth V, et al. Aluminium potroom asthma: the Norwegian experience. Eur Respir J 1994;7:165–72.
26. Desjardins A, Bergeron JP, Ghezzo H, et al. Aluminium potroom asthma confirmed by monitoring of forced expiratory volume in one second. Am J Respir Crit Care Med 1994;150:1714–7.
27. Sjåheim T, Halstensen TS, Lund MB, et al. Airway inflammation in aluminium potroom asthma. Occup Environ Med 2004;61:779–85.
28. Chan-Yeung M, Bernstein IL, Von Essen S, et al. Acute airway diseases due to organic dust exposure. In: Bernstein IL, Chan-Yeung M, Malo JL, et al, editors. Asthma in the workplace. 3rd edition. New York: Taylor & Francis; 2006. p. 641–82.
29. Cormier Y, Schuyler M. Hypersensitivity pneumonitis and organic dust toxic syndromes. In: Bernstein IL, Chan-Yeung M, Malo JL, et al, editors. Asthma in the workplace. 3rd edition. New York: Taylor & Francis Inc; 2006. p. 713–35.
30. Dolovich J, Hargreave FE. The asthma syndrome: inciters, inducers, and host characteristics. Thorax 1981;36:641–4.
31. Malo JL, Ghezzo H, L'Archevêque J, et al. Late asthmatic reactions to occupational sensitizing agents: frequency of changes in nonspecific bronchial responsiveness and of response to inhaled beta-2 adrenergic agent. J Allergy Clin Immunol 1990;85:834–42.
32. Pin I, Freitag AP, O'Byrne PM, et al. Changes in the cellular profile of induced sputum after allergen-induced asthmatic responses. Am Rev Respir Dis 1992; 145:1265–9.
33. Ihre E, Zetterstrom O. Increase in non-specific bronchial responsiveness after repeated inhalation of low doses of allergen. Clin Exp Allergy 1993;23:298–305.
34. Sulakvelidze I, Inman MD, Rerecich T, et al. Increases in airway eosinophils and interleukin-5 with minimal bronchoconstriction during repeated low-dose allergen challenge in atopic asthmatics. Eur Respir J 1998;11:821–7.
35. Malo JL, Chan-Yeung M. Agents causing occupational asthma. J Allergy Clin Immunol 2009;123:545–50.
36. Vandenplas O, Delwiche JP, Jamart J, et al. Increase in non-specific bronchial hyperresponsiveness as an early marker of bronchial response to occupational agents during specific inhalation challenges. Thorax 1996;51:472–8.
37. Lemière C, Chaboilliez S, Trudeau C, et al. Characterization of airway inflammation after repeated exposures to occupational agents. J Allergy Clin Immunol 2000;106:1163–70.
38. Brooks SM, Weiss MA, Bernstein IL. Reactive airways dysfunction syndrome (RADS). Persistent asthma syndrome after high level irritant exposures. Chest 1985;88:376–84.
39. Malo JL, L'archevêque J, Castellanos L, et al. Long-term outcomes of acute irritant-induced asthma. Am J Respir Crit Care Med 2009;179:923–8.
40. Takeda N, Maghni K, Daigle S, et al. Long-term pathologic consequences of acute irritant-induced asthma. J Allergy Clin Immunol 2009;124:975–81.
41. Harving H, Korsgaard J, Dahl R. Low concentrations of formaldehyde in bronchial asthma: a study of exposure under controlled conditions. Br Med J 1986;293:310.
42. De Luca S, Caire N, Cloutier Y, et al. Acute exposure to sawdust does not alter airway calibre and responsiveness to histamine in asthmatic subjects. Eur Respir J 1988;1:540–6.
43. Beach JR, Raven J, Ingram C, et al. The effects on asthmatics of exposure to a conventional water-based and a volatile organic compound-free paint. Eur Respir J 1997;10:563–6.

44. Committee of the Environmental and Occupational Health Assembly of the American Thoracic Society. Health effects of outdoor air pollution. Am J Respir Crit Care Med 1996;153:3–50.
45. Beach J, Rowe B, Blitz S, et al. Diagnosis and management of work-related asthma. AHRQ Publication Number 06-E003-1. Evid Rep Technol Assess (Summ) 2005;(129):1–8.
46. Vandenplas O. Socioeconomic impact of work-related asthma. Expert Rev Pharmacoecon Outcomes Res 2008;8:395–400.
47. Maestrelli P, Boschetto P, Fabbri LM, et al. Mechanisms of occupational asthma. J Allergy Clin Immunol 2009;123:531–42.
48. Koohsari H, Tamaoka M, Campbell HR, et al. The role of gamma delta T cells in airway epithelial injury and bronchial responsiveness after chlorine gas exposure in mice. Respir Res 2007;8:21–32.
49. Gautrin D, Boulet LP, Boutet M, et al. Is reactive airways dysfunction syndrome a variant of occupational asthma? J Allergy Clin Immunol 1994;93:12–22.
50. Malo JL, Cartier A, Boulet LP, et al. Bronchial hyperresponsiveness can improve while spirometry plateaus two to three years after repeated exposure to chlorine causing respiratory symptoms. Am J Respir Crit Care Med 1994;150:1142–5.
51. Gautrin D, Infante-Rivard C, Ghezzo H, et al. Incidence and host determinants of probable occupational asthma in apprentices exposed to laboratory animals. Am J Respir Crit Care Med 2001;163:899–904.
52. Chan-Yeung M, Desjardins A. Bronchial hyperresponsiveness and level of exposure in occupational asthma due to Western red cedar. Serial observations before and after development of symptoms. Am Rev Respir Dis 1992;146: 1606–9.
53. Lemière C, Cartier A, Malo JL, et al. Persistent specific bronchial reactivity to occupational agents in workers with normal nonspecific bronchial reactivity. Am J Respir Crit Care Med 2000;162:976–80.
54. Banks DE Jr, Barkman HW, Butcher BT, et al. Absence of hyperresponsiveness to methacholine in a worker with methylene diphenyl diisocyanate (MDI)-induced asthma. Chest 1986;89:389–93.
55. Thickett KM, McCoach JS, Gerber JM, et al. Occupational asthma caused by chloramines in indoor swimming-pool air. Eur Respir J 2002;19:827–32.
56. Lemière C, Weytjens K, Cartier A, et al. Late asthmatic reaction with airway inflammation but without airway hyperresponsiveness. Clin Exp Allergy 2000; 30:415–7.
57. Lemière C, D'Alpaos V, Chaboillez S, et al. Investigation of occupational asthma: sputum cell counts or exhaled nitric oxide? Chest 2010;137:617–22.
58. Leigh R, Hargreave FE. Occupational neutrophilic asthma. Can Respir J 1999;6: 194–6.
59. Lemière C, Romeo P, Chaboillez S, et al. Airway inflammation and functional changes after exposure to different concentrations of isocyanates. J Allergy Clin Immunol 2002;110:641–6.
60. Fahy JV, Liu J, Wong H, et al. Analysis of cellular and biochemical constituents of induced sputum after allergen challenge: a method for studying allergic airway inflammation. J Allergy Clin Immunol 1994;93:1031–9.
61. Stenfors N, Nordenhäll C, Salvi SS, et al. Different airway inflammatory responses in asthmatic and healthy humans exposed to diesel. Eur Respir J 2004;23:82–6.
62. Thorn J, Rylander R. Inflammatory response after inhalation of bacterial endotoxin assessed by the induced sputum technique. Thorax 1998;53:1047–52.

63. Jones KP, Mulleee MA, Middleton M, et al. Committee and the British Thoracic Society Research. Peak flow based asthma self-management: a randomised controlled study in general practice. Thorax 1995;50:851–7.
64. American Thoracic Society. Guidelines for assessing and managing asthma risk at work, school, and recreation. Am J Respir Crit Care Med 2004;169:873–81.
65. Nicholson PJ, Cullinan P, Taylor AJ, et al. Evidence based guidelines for the prevention, identification, and management of occupational asthma. Occup Environ Med 2005;62:290–9.
66. Mapp CE, Boschetto P, Maestrelli P, et al. Occupational asthma. Am J Respir Crit Care Med 2005;172:280–305.
67. Banks DE, Jalloul A. Occupational asthma, work-related asthma and reactive airways dysfunction syndrome. Curr Opin Pulm Med 2007;13:131–6.
68. Bardana EJ. Occupational asthma. J Allergy Clin Immunol 2008;121:S408–S11.
69. Dykewicz MS. Occupational asthma: current concepts in pathogenesis, diagnosis, and management. J Allergy Clin Immunol 2009;123:519–28.
70. Francis HC, Prys-Picard CO, Fishwick D, et al. Defining and investigating occupational asthma: a consensus approach. Occup Environ Med 2007;64:361–5.
71. Boulet LP. Increases in airway responsiveness following acute exposure to respiratory irritants. Reactive airway dysfunction syndrome or occupational asthma? Chest 1988;94:476–81.
72. Moore B, Sheman M. Chronic reactive airway disease following acute chlorine gas exposure in an asymptomatic atopic patient. Chest 1991;100:855.
73. Chatkin CJ, Tarlo SM, Liss G, et al. The outcome of asthma related to workplace exposures. Chest 1999;116:1780–5.
74. Chan-Yeung M, Lam S, Kennedy SM, et al. Persistent asthma after repeated exposure to high concentrations of gases in pulpmills. Am J Respir Crit Care Med 1994;149:1676–80.
75. Quirce S, Gala G, Pérez-Camo I, et al. Irritant-induced asthma: clinical and functional aspects. J Asthma 2000;37:267–74.
76. Bhérer L, Cushman R, Courteau JP, et al. Survey of construction workers repeatedly exposed to chlorine over a three to six month period in a pulpmill: II. Follow up of affected workers by questionnaire, spirometry and assessment of bronchial responsiveness 18 to 24 months after exposure. Occup Environ Med 1994;51:225–8.
77. Gautrin D, Leroyer C, Infante-Rivard C, et al. Longitudinal assessment of airway caliber and responsiveness in workers exposed to chlorine. Am J Respir Crit Care Med 1999;160:1232–7.
78. Olin AC, Andersson E, Andersson M, et al. Prevalence of asthma and exhaled nitric oxide are increased in bleachery workers exposed to ozone. Eur Respir J 2004;23:87–92.
79. Andersson E, Knutsson A, Hagberg S, et al. Incidence of asthma among workers exposed to sulphur dioxide and other irritant gases. Eur Respir J 2006;27:720–5.
80. Kogevinas M, Zock JP, Jarvis D, et al. Exposure to substances in the workplace and new-onset asthma: an international prospective population-based study (ECRHS-II). Lancet 2007;370:336–41.
81. Kipen HM, Blume R, Hutt D. Asthma experience in an occupational and environmental medicine clinic. Low-dose reactive airways dysfunction syndrome. J Occup Med 1994;36:1133–7.
82. Brooks SM, Hammad Y, Richards I, et al. The spectrum of irritant-induced asthma. Chest 1998;113:42–9.

83. Chan-Yeung M. Occupational asthma—the past 50 years. Can Respir J 2004; 11:21–6.
84. Malo JL, Ghezzo H, L'Archevêque J, et al. Is the clinical history a satisfactory means of diagnosing occupational asthma? Am Rev Respir Dis 1991;143: 528–32.
85. Tarlo SM, Leung K, Broder I, et al. Asthmatic subjects symptomatically worse at work: prevalence and characterization among a general asthma clinic population. Chest 2000;118:1309–14.
86. Vandenplas O, Ghezzo H, Munoz X, et al. What are the questionnaire items most useful in identifying subjects with occupational asthma? Eur Respir J 2005;26: 1056–63.
87. Larbanois A, Jamart J, Delwiche JP, et al. Socioeconomic outcome of subjects experiencing asthma symptoms at work. Eur Respir J 2002;19:1107–13.
88. Lemière C, Pelissier S, Chaboillez S, et al. Outcome of subjects diagnosed with occupational asthma and work-aggravated asthma after removal from exposure. J Occup Environ Med 2006;48:656–9.
89. Chiry S, Cartier A, Malo JL, et al. Comparison of peak expiratory flow variability between workers with work-exacerbated asthma and occupational asthma. Chest 2007;132:483–8.
90. Santos MS, Jung H, Peyrovi J, et al. Occupational asthma and work-exacerbated asthma: factors associated with time to diagnostic steps. Chest 2007;131(6):1768–75.
91. Girard F, Chaboillez S, Cartier A, et al. An effective strategy for diagnosing occupational asthma. Induced sputum. Am J Respir Crit Care Med 2004;170:845–50.
92. Vandenplas O, D'Alpaos V, Heymans J, et al. Sputum eosinophilia: an early marker of bronchial response to occupational agents. Allergy 2009;64:754–61.
93. Lemiere C, Forget A, Dufour MH, et al. Characteristics and medical resource use of asthmatic subjects with and without work-related asthma. J Allergy Clin Immunol 2007;120:1354–9.
94. Curwick CC, Bonauto DK, Adams DA. Use of objective testing in the diagnosis of work-related asthma by physician specialty. Ann Allergy Asthma Immunol 2006;97:546–50.
95. Fishwick D, Bradshaw L, Davies J, et al. Are we failing workers with symptoms suggestive of occupational asthma? Prim Care Respir J 2007;16:304–10.
96. Vandenplas O, Toren K, Blanc P. Health and socioeconomic impact of work-related asthma. Eur Respir J 2003;22:689–97.
97. Jajosky RA, Harrison R, Reinisch F, et al. Surveillance of work-related asthma in selected U.S. states using surveillance guidelines for state health departments—California, Massachusetts, Michigan and New Jersey. MMWR CDC Surveill Summ 1999;48(SS-3):1–20.
98. Chan-Yeung M. Assessment of asthma in the workplace. Chest 1995;108: 1084–117.
99. Chan-Yeung M, Malo JL. Occupational asthma. N Engl J Med 1995;333:107–12.
100. Beach J, Russell K, Blitz S, et al. A systematic review of the diagnosis of occupational asthma. Chest 2007;131:569–78.

The Epidemiology of Work-Related Asthma

Andrew M. Smith, MD, MS[a,b,*]

KEYWORDS

• Asthma • Workplace • Epidemiology • Bronchospasm

Work-related asthma has been used to describe all asthmatic conditions related to workplace exposures, such as:

1. Occupational asthma, which is induced by sensitizers or irritants at work
2. Work-exacerbated asthma, bronchospasm provoked by triggers and work in workers with preexisting asthma.[1,2]

Both conditions may coexist in the same patient and are not mutually exclusive.

Occupational asthma is defined as pulmonary disease characterized by airway hyperresponsiveness, variable airflow limitation, and inflammation attributable to an occupational environment and not to exposures encountered outside the workplace.[3] There are 2 distinct subtypes of occupational asthma. The first is work-related asthma caused by either reactive chemical sensitizers or natural protein allergens after a latency period of exposure. The second is irritant-induced asthma, which has no preceding latency, no history of preexisting asthma, and occurs after single or multiple exposures to high levels of irritants at work.

Respiratory sensitizers, such as natural proteins or low-molecular-weight reactive chemicals acting as haptens, may induce occupational asthma through immunoglobulin E (IgE)–dependent mechanisms. Although immunologic mechanisms are suspected for many causative chemical sensitizers, these are not always associated with demonstrable, specific IgE responses.[4]

Reactive airways dysfunction syndrome is the best-defined phenotype of irritant-induced asthma. This syndrome is characterized by acute respiratory symptoms, such as cough, dyspnea, and/or wheezing, starting within 24 hours from a single, high-level exposure to a workplace irritant.[5,6] If the onset of symptoms is greater than 24 hours after multiple irritant exposures, the term irritant-induced asthma is used.[5]

Work-exacerbated asthma, bronchospasm triggered at work, can be worsened by intermittent exposure to chemical fumes such as bleach among cleaning workers,

[a] Department of Internal Medicine, Division of Immunology, University of Cincinnati, 3255 Eden Avenue, ML 0563, Cincinnati, OH 45267-0563, USA
[b] Allergy Section, Cincinnati VA Medical Center, 3200 Vine Street, Cincinnati, OH 45220, USA
* Department of Internal Medicine, Division of Immunology, University of Cincinnati, 3255 Eden Avenue, ML 0563, Cincinnati, OH 45267-0563.
E-mail address: Andrew.Smith@uc.edu

Immunol Allergy Clin N Am 31 (2011) 663–675
doi:10.1016/j.iac.2011.07.009
0889-8561/11/$ – see front matter © 2011 Elsevier Inc. All rights reserved.

and other chemical fumes such as sulfur dioxide, chlorine gas, and environmental tobacco smoke.[7,8]

Given the breadth of phenotypes and exposures that can be associated with work-related asthma, this article addresses the epidemiology of occupational asthma and work-exacerbated asthma by the individual environmental exposures that commonly are associated with these disorders.

ESTABLISHING AN OBJECTIVE DIAGNOSIS OF WORK-RELATED ASTHMA

An accurate estimation of the epidemiology of work-related asthma depends on the accurate characterization and diagnosis of work-related asthma phenotypes. The diagnostic methods for occupational asthma and work-exacerbated asthma have been reviewed elsewhere.[9–11] The diagnosis should not be based on medical history alone without objective confirmation by measurements of lung function at work and away from work.[12] Failure to establish an accurate diagnosis could allow for miscategorization of the occupational asthma phenotype and inaccurate estimates of incidence and prevalence.

There are 3 major components in the current diagnostic approach for work-related asthma. The first is obtaining a compatible occupational and medical history. The second is confirming an objective diagnosis of asthma. The third is showing decrements in lung function when exposed to conditions or substances at work, along with improvement for sufficient time away from work. A published list of agents known to cause occupational asthma can be researched as well (www.asmanet.com). Of the approximately 400 known causes of occupational asthma, most are high-molecular-weight protein sensitizers, whereas fewer than 30 are low-molecular-weight agents or reactive chemicals. If possible, skin testing or in vitro serologic testing can be used to confirm clinically relevant respiratory sensitizers from the workplace.[11] As part of the evaluation, conditions that could mimic work-related asthma, such as vocal cord dysfunction, which can be triggered by workplace exposures, should be excluded.[13]

EPIDEMIOLOGY OF WORK-RELATED ASTHMA BY EXPOSURE

The exact incidence and prevalence of work-related asthma are not well defined. It is estimated that 10% to 25% of adult cases of asthma are aggravated by occupational factors.[14–16] In a 15-year surveillance study, the annual incidence of occupational asthma was 42 (95% confidence interval [CI] 37–45) per million working population (**Fig. 1**).[17] Of all workers identified with work-related asthma, work-exacerbated asthma cases may represent between 10% and 50%.[18,19] It is likely that

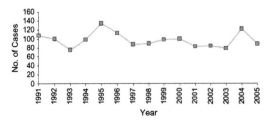

Fig. 1. Incidence of occupational asthma. Number of new cases reported annually to Shield from 1991 to 2005. (*From* Bakerly ND, Moore VC, Vellore AD, et al. Fifteen-year trends in occupational asthma: data from the Shield surveillance scheme. Occup Med (Lond) 2008;58(3):170; with permission.)

work-exacerbated asthma is highly prevalent and underdiagnosed, given that an estimated 18% of the global population is affected by asthma.[20]

DIISOCYANATE

The diisocyanates are a family of highly reactive, low-molecular-weight chemicals, including hexamethylene diisocyanate (HDI), methylene diphenyl diisocyanate (MDI), and toluene diisocyanate (TDI). Among workers, there is extensive exposure to diisocyanates. More than 253,000 US workers in the transportation industries are employed in facilities that use isocyanates.[21] Other industries with diisocyanate exposure include spray painting, particularly automobile repair (HDI), manufacture of polyurethane foam (MDI), manufacture of particle board (MDI), use in foundries (MDI), and manufacture of polyurethane foam (TDI).

The main route of occupational exposure is through inhalation. Inhalation of diisocyanate fumes is associated with various pulmonary diseases, such as occupational asthma, hypersensitivity pneumonitis and direct toxic effects.[22–26] Diisocyanates are potent sensitizers, and have long been recognized as a cause of occupational disease, particularly asthma.[23,27–29] The degree of exposure directly affects the prevalence and incidence of diisocyanate-induced conditions. On average, numerous studies have documented that 5% to 15% of those who work with diisocyanates develop occupational asthma, making this the most common cause of occupational asthma (**Fig. 2**).[26]

The incidence and prevalence of diisocyanate asthma can be affected by avoidance and industrial hygiene measures. Negative pressure, air-purifying, half-facepiece respirators using prefilters and organic vapor cartridges have been reported to provide effective protection for spray painters exposed to diisocyanates.[30] Despite industrial hygiene measures that maintain ambient chemical exposures in a factory at less than threshold limit values, incident cases of occupational asthma still occur.[31] In the case of diisocyanate chemicals, new cases of occupational asthma may develop after intermittent accidental chemical exposures during maintenance procedures or from accidental spills of MDI or TDI, when exposure may escape detection by continuous monitors.

NATURAL RUBBER LATEX

Natural rubber latex (NRL) is a complex mixture of at least 13 allergenic proteins that bind human IgE antibodies (Hev b allergens), derived from the sap of the rubber tree, *Hevea brasiliensis*.[32] Through the use of NRL gloves, health care workers are commonly exposed to Hev b allergens in an occupational setting.

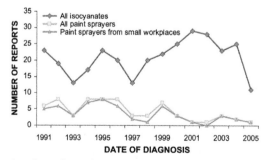

Fig. 2. Occupational asthma from diisocyanates. Total numbers of occupational asthma cases from isocyanates per year for 15 years by job category. (*From* Bakerly ND, Moore VC, Vellore AD, et al. Fifteen-year trends in occupational asthma: data from the Shield surveillance scheme. Occup Med (Lond) 2008;58(3):171; with permission.)

Among health care workers who use NRL gloves, occupational asthma as a result of exposure increased significantly during the 1990s (**Fig. 3**). Several studies have evaluated the long-term changes in occupational asthma with changes in NRL glove use. In a survey of 332 health care workers, 20 (6%) reported new-onset asthma in a 9-year period.[33] Compared with controls, hospital technicians had a significant increased risk of asthma (rate ratio [RR] 4.63; 95% CI 1.87–11.5). In a 15-year occupational asthma surveillance study, 1461 cases were reported.[17] Of these cases, 85% had a confirmatory test for asthma. Health care workers accounted for 125 cases (9%) of incident occupational asthma. Latex was implicated as the causative agent in 91 (6% of the total incident cases). With the change to latex-free or low-protein, powder-free latex gloves, there was a significant reduction in incidence in the last 2 years of the surveillance. Another estimate of the incidence of occupational asthma from NRL comes from a retrospective review of occupational claims among health care workers from 1982 to 2004.[34] Of the 298 cases reviewed, 127 were categorized as definite NRL occupational asthma and 68 as probable NRL occupational asthma. This study also reported a significant decrease in the incidence of NRL occupational asthma among health care workers from 1999 onwards with changes away from powdered NRL gloves.

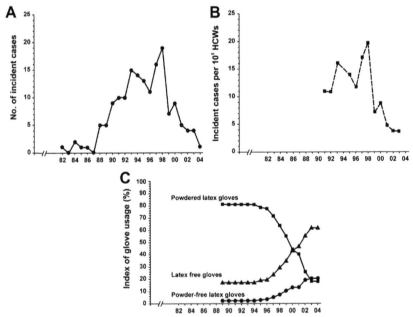

Fig. 3. Occupational asthma from NRL. (*A*) Annual numbers of definite and probable cases of NRL-induced occupational asthma in health care workers categorized by the year of the onset of work-related asthma symptoms. (*B*) Incidence rates of NRL-induced occupational asthma expressed as the number of incident cases per 10^5 full-time equivalents of nonadministrative employees in Belgian hospitals. (*C*) Usage indices (expressed as percentage of total glove usage) of the different types of gloves in surveyed Belgian hospitals rectangles, powdered latex gloves; triangles, latex-free gloves; circles, powder-free latex gloves). HCWs, health care workers. (*From* Vandenplas O, Larbanois A, Vanassche F, et al. Latex-induced occupational asthma: time trend in incidence and relationship with hospital glove policies. Allergy 2009;64(3):418; with permission.)

WHEAT FLOUR

The prevalence of bakers' asthma among bakery employees exposed to wheat flour is estimated to be 9%.[35] In one study, 139 workers who were occupationally exposed to wheat flour were evaluated.[35] Of these workers, 30 were found to have asthma along with either a positive skin prick test to crude wheat flour extract or an increased in vitro specific IgE to wheat flour.

Surveillance for asthma symptoms among bakery workers is an important means to detect early disease. In 1 study, the spirometric measurements of 58 bakery workers were compared with those of 45 nonbakers.[36] There was a statistically significant difference between bakery workers and controls for baseline mean forced expiratory volume in the first second of expiration (FEV_1) percent predicted (91.6 vs 101.7) and mean forced vital capacity (FVC) percent predicted (94.5 vs 99.9). None of the controls had an obstructive defect (FEV_1/FVC ratio $\leq$ lower limit of normal) compared with 12.1% of bakery workers. Another study evaluated the role of exposure to wheat in the development of occupational disease among 860 bakers.[37] Both atopy and sensitization to wheat flour were found to be risk factors for the development of work-related asthma. The prevalence of work-related asthma was significantly higher among bakers sensitized to wheat flour (35% among sensitized vs 6% among nonsensitized) and among bakers with other atopic disease (42% among atopic sensitized vs 11% among atopic nonsensitized). A further study found a lower rate specifically of bakers' asthma among 392 bakers.[38] Among the bakers, 17.1% of workers complained of respiratory symptoms. Specific inhalation challenge with wheat flour extracts confirmed bakers' asthma among 1.5% of the baker population studied.

ANIMAL ALLERGY (MAMMALIAN PROTEINS)

Among laboratory animal workers, allergic reactions are an important occupational health problem, with an estimated incidence of 1.32 per 100 person years and an estimated prevalence of 22% in this environment.[39] Veterinarians are at the highest risk of developing work-related asthma of all animal workers. Early work compared the occurrence of respiratory disease between 257 veterinarians and 100 controls.[40] The prevalence of asthma was higher among the veterinarians (16.3%) compared with controls (6%) (P<.05). Only 6 veterinarians reported asthma symptoms related to animal exposure. A larger study of 1416 veterinarians found a higher rate of work-related asthma.[39] Among these veterinarians, 20% reported asthma symptoms in the work environment. Cats were the most commonly reported animals causing work-related symptoms in 58% of affected workers, with dogs causing symptoms in 31%. A further study investigated the risk factors for occupational asthma among 200 veterinarians working with laboratory animals. Chest symptoms were reported in 19 (9.5%) of workers. Of those veterinarians sensitized to laboratory animals by skin testing or specific IgE testing, 14 (11.4%) reported chest symptoms at work. In addition to cat sensitization (odds ratio [OR] 10.27; 95% CI 2.42–49.91), daily contact with laboratory animals (OR 4.52; 95% CI 1.53–13.73) (rat, mouse, hamster, guinea pig, rabbit), and working time of more than 10 years (OR 5.21; 95% CI 1.37–29.10) were found to be significant risk factors for the development of occupational asthma.

SEAFOOD/SEA SQUIRT

Employment associated with the seafood industry is common, with 43 million people worldwide reported as workers in the industry.[41] A variety of work activities can lead to significant exposure to seafood, such as the harvesting of seafood, processing of seafood in factories, food preparation, and laboratory exposure. Common agents causing occupational asthma include the crustaceans (eg, crab, lobsters, shrimp), the mollusks (eg, clams, oysters, mussels, scallops), bony fish such as salmon and tuna, and other associated biologic agents, such as sea squirt.[42] Seafood contains a wide variety of proteins. Of these, many seafood allergens have been identified, including tropomysin and parvalbumin. Across the seafood industry, prevalence estimates of occupational asthma range from 2% to 36%.[43] The estimates of disease burden critically depend on the definition of disease, the type of work performed, and the allergenicity of seafood exposure. An updated review of reports of occupational asthma across the seafood industry has recently been published.[43]

Asthma caused by exposure to sea squirt allergens primarily occurs among Japanese oyster shucking workers. The major allergens are from the body fluid of the sea squirt, *Styela plicata*, and are the acidic glycoproteins, Gi-rep, Ei-M, and DIIIa. Oyster shucking workers constantly inhale the sea squirt antigens in the mist of the body fluid of sea squirts while at work. The reported prevalence of sea squirt asthma among oyster shucking workers was 36% in 1963.[44] This significant prevalence has dramatically decreased with industrial hygiene improvements. A more recently reported prevalence of sea squirt asthma has decreased to 8%, with an incidence of 10.1% among oyster shucking workers.[44]

HOUSE-DUST MITE AND DOMESTIC/NONDOMESTIC CLEANING

House-dust mite is the most common indoor allergen.[45] In rooms with wall-to-wall carpeting, high levels of the allergens of house-dust mite species *Dermatophagoides pteronyssinus* (Der p1) and *Dermatophagoides farinae* (Der f1) are present in the house dust. In a variety of occupations, such as domestic cleaners and janitorial staff, exposure to house-dust mite allergens (Der p1 and Der f1) is unavoidable. However, as part of the occupation, chemical and irritant exposure is also common.

To evaluate the risks of work-related asthma among domestic and nondomestic cleaners, several studies have been performed. In a cross-sectional study, 4521 women were evaluated.[46] Among the cleaners, the prevalence of asthma and work-related respiratory symptoms was 12%. Compared with noncleaners, the cleaners had a significant increased risk of asthma (OR 1.46; 95% CI 1.10–1.92). Another study followed 43 female domestic cleaners, with data gathered through a 2-week diary.[7] Although vacuuming and house dust mite exposure was associated with upper respiratory symptoms (OR 2.0; 95% CI 1.0–4.2), this exposure was not associated with work-related asthma. Instead, cleaning product exposure (bleach, ammonia, air freshener) was associated with work-related asthma in 30% of the cleaners. A further study evaluated 1500 cleaners, both men and women.[47] In this study, work-related asthma symptoms were significantly associated with waxing floors, cleaning bathrooms, spot-cleaning carpet, and oiling furniture (all irritant exposures). Based on available data, it is possible that house dust mite exposure may play a role in work-related asthma, but, to date, irritant exposures seem to play a more significant role among cleaners.

DETERGENT

In the 1960s, alkaline-stable and heat-stable proteolytic enzymes were introduced into detergents to improve the performance of the detergent. Allergic reactions, particularly occupational asthma, to the proteolytic enzymes in detergent products were first reported in 1969.[48,49] The risk of allergic antibody-mediated occupational asthma caused by enzyme use in the detergent industry was quickly recognized. In a 20-year study, the lung function in 731 workers exposed to proteolytic enzymes derived from *Bacillus* species in the 5 detergent factories was evaluated.[50] During the study period, 166 cases of enzyme asthma were confirmed among workers. In a 10-year continuing surveillance study, several thousand workers were tracked for the development of occupational asthma after the continued use of industrial hygiene measures to decrease exposure to the proteolytic enzymes (**Fig. 4**).[51] In the study period, only 17 cases of occupational asthma were confirmed among the workers.

ACID ANHYDRIDE CHEMICALS

There are rare chemical sensitizers shown to cause occupational asthma through specific IgE mechanisms. Acid anhydride chemicals (eg, trimellitic anhydride, phthalic anhydride), which represent the prototypic class of reactive chemical haptens, can form allergenic determinants by combining with autologous respiratory proteins in vivo.

A study of 27 workers with exposure to hexahydrophthalic anhydride (HHPA) from an epoxy resin molding system was performed to evaluate the nature of respiratory complaints. For each worker, estimates of exposure were made from both job description and environmental sampling. Seven workers (25.9%) reported symptoms of asthma and rhinitis. Four workers had symptoms consistent with occupational asthma (14.8%). None of the workers showed a significant preshift-to-postshift decrease in FEV_1. The overall prevalence of work-related asthma based on these data is 40.7%.

In another group of workers exposed to hexahydrophthalic anhydride for manufacturing an epoxy resin product, the effect of respiratory protective devices was evaluated. For the 7-year study, 66 workers were followed.[52] With the use of respiratory protective devices, an estimated 80% reduction in the expected incidence of occupational respiratory disease was reported. However, this preventive measure did not prevent 3 new cases of occupational asthma. During the study, the incidence per year of occupational asthma related to HHPA exposure dropped from 10% to 2% and the prevalence decreased from 7.5% to less than 1%.

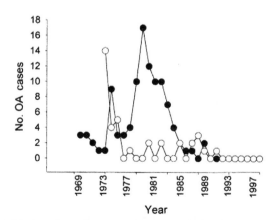

Fig. 4. Occupational asthma from detergent enzymes. Number of occupational asthma cases per year at all Latin American (filled circle) and North American (empty circle) enzyme-detergent manufacturing sites (1969–1998). (*From* Schweigert MK, Mackenzie DP, Sarlo K. Occupational asthma and allergy associated with the use of enzymes in the detergent industry–a review of the epidemiology, toxicology and methods of prevention. Clin Exp Allergy 2000;30(11):1512; with permission.)

IRRITANTS

It is estimated that 25 million workers are exposed to environmental tobacco smoke (ETS) at work.[53] The impact of various asthma triggers encountered on the job (eg, ETS, aeroallergens, exertion, and irritants) and their overall impact on the asthma disease burden is unknown. Data regarding the impact of occupational ETS exposure on work-related asthma have been provided in a prospective cohort study of 77 bar workers evaluated before and after institution of a cigarette smoking ban. The cigarette smoking ban effectively eliminated the workers' exposures to secondhand ETS. In a subset of 10 of 77 workers with preexisting asthma, there was a 10% increase in mean FEV_1 and a significant improvement in quality of life measures after institution of the smoking ban.[8] Most recently, an evaluation of the impact of a 100% smoke-free workplace legislation among hospitality workers in Argentina was reported.[54] In 2007, a ban on cigarette smoking in public venues and workplaces was enacted. Surveys and spirometric measurements were performed before and after the smoking ban. From 101 bars and restaurants, 80 workers completed the full evaluation. There was a significant reduction in reported respiratory symptoms (cough, wheezing, dyspnea, and chest tightness) from 58% of workers before the ban to 29% or workers after the ban. However, no significant change in FEV_1 was seen.

Another irritant exposure that has been studied is exposure to chlorine and halogenated disinfection by-products (DBPs) among workers at indoor pools. High rates of respiratory symptoms suggesting asthma have been reported in several epidemiologic studies.[37,55–57] Of 334 lifeguards, 3 of 83 with the highest exposure to DBPs (3.6%) reported occupational asthma symptoms.[55] In a case series of 3 pool workers with occupational symptoms, work-related asthma was confirmed by workplace challenge.[57] Two of the workers reported preexisting asthma, making their diagnosis work-exacerbated asthma. In a cross-sectional survey of 624 pool workers in whom asthma symptoms were assessed by questionnaire, asthma symptoms were significantly increased compared with a population control sample (OR range 1.4–7.2).[37] In the most recent study, the prevalence of work-related asthma was assessed with 133 pool workers in a cross-sectional study.[58] A prevalence of asthma was reported as 7.5% across all workers (high and low exposure). However, there was a significant increase in work-related asthma among those workers with high exposure (OR 5.1; 95% CI 1.0–27.2).

PREVENTION OF WORK-RELATED ASTHMA
Primary Prevention

Incident cases of occupational asthma provide a unique opportunity to identify a high-risk work environment and to advise an employer to enact control measures that may prevent new cases among similarly exposed workers (primary prevention). Ideally, prevention of new cases could be achieved if threshold exposure limits could be defined below which the development of occupational asthma is unlikely.[59] Interventions may include substituting a safer alternative substance for the causative agent in the industrial process. Because this is often not feasible, substantial reduction in human exposure to causative chemicals may be achieved through the introduction of new engineering controls, which may prevent new cases of occupational asthma.

Understanding of the periods of risk from exposure is also important. In a recent long-term prospective cohort study, the highest incidence of bronchial hyperresponsiveness among apprentice laboratory animal workers exposed to high-molecular-weight antigens was exhibited in the first years of work. This finding might indicate a time at which increased control of exposure might modify risk.[60]

Effective primary prevention has been shown by the successful control of occupational asthma achieved in health care workers exposed to NRL gloves. Powdered NRL gloves were substituted with powder-free NRL gloves and/or low-protein powder-free NRL gloves in 8 primary prevention programs among health care worker populations. This substitution resulted in reduced levels of ambient measurable NRL aeroallergens and decreased incident cases of occupational asthma among the previously exposed health care workers.[61]

Industrial hygiene programs in the detergent manufacturing industry are another example of successful primary prevention of occupational asthma. The specific measures include (1) encapsulation of detergent enzyme protein granules in inert materials; (2) frequent ambient monitoring for enzymatic proteins; (3) engineering controls to minimize ambient enzyme dust; and (4) employee training to minimize personal exposure. These approaches have been used to maintain ambient enzyme levels at less than 15 ng protein/m^3 (less than the ACGIH TLV of 60 ng protein/m^3). This decreased exposure had resulted in dramatic declines in detergent enzyme sensitization rates and incident cases of occupational asthma.[51]

As an example of substitution, diisocyanates, previously used in monomeric forms as paint hardeners or for urethane production, are now sold almost entirely as prepolymerized products (polyisocyanates), likely reducing respiratory and dermal exposure to active diisocyanate molecules. As an example of new engineering controls in most modern plants, spray painting of hard metal surfaces using hexamethylene diisocyanate, an essential paint hardener, is performed by robotic devices enclosed in independently ventilated paint booths. It is thought that, in diisocyanate-exposed workers, these measures may have reduced new cases of occupational asthma.

Secondary Prevention

Early identification of workers with occupational symptoms, such as occupational allergic rhinitis, followed by significant reduction in occupational exposure, may prevent incident cases of occupational asthma (secondary prevention). As an example, the detergent enzyme industry has instituted exemplary medical surveillance programs. Surveillance is conducted annually among exposed workers through medical questionnaires and skin testing with enzyme solutions (such as *Aspergillus*-derived amylase and *Bacillus subtilis* protease).[51] If a sensitized worker develops allergic rhinitis symptoms, the worker is relocated away from potential high-exposure areas. In one detergent company, the annual incidence of newly sensitized workers was maintained at less than 3% with no incident occupational asthma cases reported in a 6-year period after the establishment of surveillance and industrial hygiene programs.[51]

Tertiary Prevention

Specific methods of environmental control of harmful exposures, such as removing a worker with established occupational asthma from exposure to a newly recognized occupational sensitizer, must be personalized to the specific needs of each worker with occupational asthma (tertiary prevention). In the case of a worker with preexisting occupational asthma, efforts are directed at preventing progression to more severe asthma along with the progressive loss in lung function caused by the continued exposure to offending agents at work. This approach to tertiary prevention is supported by a recent retrospective study of more than 150 consecutive cases of occupational asthma. Workers removed from occupational exposure showed a decelerated rate of decline in FEV_1 in 6 months or more after the removal of the exposure.[62]

SUMMARY

Much has been learned from epidemiologic studies conducted in the past 4 decades that can be directly applied to the management of workers affected with occupational asthma. The workplace is an ever-changing environment that offers unique opportunities to investigate the natural history of work-related asthma. Past investigations have provided invaluable information about host factors in workers as well as environmental exposure characteristics that may enhance disease susceptibility. Longitudinal studies have characterized those occupational agents posing the highest risks (eg, low-molecular-weight chemicals such as diisocyanates) for development of severe irreversible airway obstruction and asthma disability from occupational asthma, especially when exposure is continued after the diagnosis is established.

Identification of sentinel cases of occupational asthma have enabled investigators to develop methods for screening workers at risk and novel interventions that may prevent new cases among exposed worker populations. Primary prevention efforts including workplace exposure modification and product modifications have, in certain cases, virtually eliminated new cases of occupational asthma caused by specific sensitizers (eg, NRL). Less is known about the natural history and chronic morbidity associated with work-aggravated asthma and irritant-induced asthma syndromes; more studies are needed in at-risk worker populations.

REFERENCES

1. Breton CV, Zhang Z, Hunt PR, et al. Characteristics of work related asthma: results from a population based survey. Occup Environ Med 2006;63(6):411–5.
2. Henneberger PK, Derk SJ, Sama SR, et al. The frequency of workplace exacerbation among health maintenance organisation members with asthma. Occup Environ Med 2006;63(8):551–7.
3. Bernstein IL. Asthma in the workplace, and related conditions. New York: Taylor & Francis; 2006.
4. Bernstein DI, Cartier A, Côté J, et al. Diisocyanate antigen-stimulated monocyte chemoattractant protein-1 synthesis has greater test efficiency than specific antibodies for identification of diisocyanate asthma. Am J Respir Crit Care Med 2002; 166(4):445–50.
5. Brooks SM, Hammad Y, Richards I, et al. The spectrum of irritant-induced asthma: sudden and not-so-sudden onset and the role of allergy. Chest 1998; 113(1):42–9.
6. Brooks SM, Weiss MA, Bernstein IL. Reactive airways dysfunction syndrome (RADS). Persistent asthma syndrome after high level irritant exposures. Chest 1985;88(3):376–84.
7. Medina-Ramon M, Zock JP, Kogevinas M, et al. Short-term respiratory effects of cleaning exposures in female domestic cleaners. Eur Respir J 2006;27(6): 1196–203.
8. Menzies D, Nair A, Williamson PA, et al. Respiratory symptoms, pulmonary function, and markers of inflammation among bar workers before and after a legislative ban on smoking in public places. JAMA 2006;296(14):1742–8.
9. Newman Taylor AJ, Cullinan P, Burge PS, et al. BOHRF guidelines for occupational asthma. Thorax 2005;60(5):364–6.
10. Nicholson PJ, Cullinan P, Taylor AJ, et al. Evidence based guidelines for the prevention, identification, and management of occupational asthma. Occup Environ Med 2005;62(5):290–9.

11. Tarlo SM, Balmes J, Balkissoon R, et al. Diagnosis and management of work-related asthma: American College Of Chest Physicians Consensus Statement. Chest 2008;134(Suppl 3):1S–41S.
12. Malo JL, Ghezzo H, L'Archevêque J, et al. Is the clinical history a satisfactory means of diagnosing occupational asthma? Am Rev Respir Dis 1991;143(3):528–32.
13. Perkner JJ, Fennelly KP, Balkissoon R, et al. Irritant-associated vocal cord dysfunction. J Occup Environ Med 1998;40(2):136–43.
14. Balmes J, Becklake M, Blanc P, et al. American Thoracic Society Statement: occupational contribution to the burden of airway disease. Am J Respir Crit Care Med 2003;167(5):787–97.
15. Blanc PD, Toren K. How much adult asthma can be attributed to occupational factors? Am J Med 1999;107(6):580–7.
16. Kogevinas M, Zock JP, Jarvis D, et al. Exposure to substances in the workplace and new-onset asthma: an international prospective population-based study (ECRHS-II). Lancet 2007;370(9584):336–41.
17. Bakerly ND, Moore VC, Vellore AD, et al. Fifteen-year trends in occupational asthma: data from the Shield surveillance scheme. Occup Med (Lond) 2008; 58(3):169–74.
18. Goe SK, Henneberger PK, Reilly MJ, et al. A descriptive study of work aggravated asthma. Occup Environ Med 2004;61(6):512–7.
19. Rosenman KD, Reilly MJ, Kalinowski DJ. A state-based surveillance system for work-related asthma. J Occup Environ Med 1997;39(5):415–25.
20. Bateman ED, Hurd SS, Barnes PJ, et al. Global strategy for asthma management and prevention: GINA executive summary. Eur Respir J 2008;31(1):143–78.
21. Alert: preventing asthma and death from MDI exposure during spray-on truck bed liner and related applications. NIOSH Publication 2006-149. Cincinnati (OH): NIOSH; 2006. p. 1–42.
22. Baur X. New aspects of isocyanate asthma. Lung 1990;168(Suppl):606–13.
23. Karol MH. Respiratory effects of inhaled isocyanates. Crit Rev Toxicol 1986;16(4): 349–79.
24. Kennedy AL, Brown WE. Isocyanates and lung disease: experimental approaches to molecular mechanisms. Occup Med 1992;7(2):301–29.
25. Mapp CE, Saetta M, Maestrelli P, et al. Low molecular weight pollutants and asthma: pathogenetic mechanisms and genetic factors. Eur Respir J 1994;7(9): 1559–63.
26. Redlich CA, Karol MH. Diisocyanate asthma: clinical aspects and immunopathogenesis. Int Immunopharmacol 2002;2(2–3):213–24.
27. Baur X, Marek W, Ammon J, et al. Respiratory and other hazards of isocyanates. Int Arch Occup Environ Health 1994;66(3):141–52.
28. Bernstein JA. Overview of diisocyanate occupational asthma. Toxicology 1996; 111(1–3):181–9.
29. A summary of health hazard evaluations: issues related to occupational exposure to isocyanates, 1989 to 2002. DHHS (NIOSH) Publication No. 2004-116. Cincinnati (OH): NIOSH; 2004. p. 1–42.
30. Liu Y, Stowe MH, Bello D, et al. Respiratory protection from isocyanate exposure in the autobody repair and refinishing industry. J Occup Environ Hyg 2006;3(5): 234–49.
31. Bernstein DI, Korbee L, Stauder T, et al. The low prevalence of occupational asthma and antibody-dependent sensitization to diphenylmethane diisocyanate in a plant engineered for minimal exposure to diisocyanates. J Allergy Clin Immunol 1993;92(3):387–96.

32. Sussman GL, Beezhold DH, Liss G. Latex allergy: historical perspective. Methods 2002;27(1):3–9.
33. Mirabelli MC, Zock JP, Plana E, et al. Occupational risk factors for asthma among nurses and related healthcare professionals in an international study. Occup Environ Med 2007;64(7):474–9.
34. Vandenplas O, Larbanois A, Vanassche F, et al. Latex-induced occupational asthma: time trend in incidence and relationship with hospital glove policies. Allergy 2009;64(3):415–20.
35. Armentia A, Martin-Santos JM, Quintero A, et al. Bakers' asthma: prevalence and evaluation of immunotherapy with a wheat flour extract. Ann Allergy 1990;65(4): 265–72.
36. Patouchas D, Efremidis G, Karkoulias K, et al. Lung function measurements in traditional bakers. Acta Biomed 2008;79(3):197–203.
37. Jacobs JH, Spaan S, van Rooy GB, et al. Exposure to trichloramine and respiratory symptoms in indoor swimming pool workers. Eur Respir J 2007;29(4):690–8.
38. Hur GY, Koh DH, Kim HA, et al. Prevalence of work-related symptoms and serum-specific antibodies to wheat flour in exposed workers in the bakery industry. Respir Med 2008;102(4):548–55.
39. Susitaival P, Kirk JH, Schenker MB. Atopic symptoms among California veterinarians. Am J Ind Med 2003;44(2):166–71.
40. Lutsky I, Baum GL, Teichtahl H, et al. Occupational respiratory disease in veterinarians. Ann Allergy 1985;55(2):153–6.
41. Food and Agriculture Organization of the United Nations. Fisheries Dept. The state of world fisheries and aquaculture. Rome (Italy): Food and Agriculture Organization of the United Nations; 2009. p. v.
42. Jeebhay MF, Robins TG, Lehrer SB, et al. Occupational seafood allergy: a review. Occup Environ Med 2001;58(9):553–62.
43. Jeebhay MF, Cartier A. Seafood workers and respiratory disease: an update. Curr Opin Allergy Clin Immunol 2010;10(2):104–13.
44. Ohtsuka T, Tsuboi S, Katsutani T, et al. [Results of 29-year study of hoya (sea-squirt) asthma in Hatsukaichi, Hiroshima prefecture]. Arerugi 1993;42(3 Pt 1): 214–8 [in Japanese].
45. Platts-Mills TA, Vervloet D, Thomas WR, et al. Indoor allergens and asthma: report of the Third International Workshop. J Allergy Clin Immunol 1997;100(6 Pt 1): S2–24.
46. Medina-Ramon M, Zock JP, Kogevinas M, et al. Asthma symptoms in women employed in domestic cleaning: a community based study. Thorax 2003;58(11): 950–4.
47. Obadia M, Liss GM, Lou W, et al. Relationships between asthma and work exposures among non-domestic cleaners in Ontario. Am J Ind Med 2009;52(9): 716–23.
48. Flindt ML. Pulmonary disease due to inhalation of derivatives of Bacillus subtilis containing proteolytic enzyme. Lancet 1969;1(7607):1177–81.
49. Pepys J, Longbottom JL, Hargreave FE, et al. Allergic reactions of the lungs to enzymes of Bacillus subtilis. Lancet 1969;1(7607):1181–4.
50. Cathcart M, Nicholson P, Roberts D, et al. Enzyme exposure, smoking and lung function in employees in the detergent industry over 20 years. Medical Subcommittee of the UK Soap and Detergent Industry Association. Occup Med (Lond) 1997;47(8):473–8.
51. Schweigert MK, Mackenzie DP, Sarlo K. Occupational asthma and allergy associated with the use of enzymes in the detergent industry–a review of the

epidemiology, toxicology and methods of prevention. Clin Exp Allergy 2000; 30(11):1511–8.

52. Grammer LC, Harris KE, et al. Effect of respiratory protective devices on development of antibody and occupational asthma to an acid anhydride. Chest 2002;121(4):1317–22.

53. Jaakkola MS, Jaakkola JJ. Impact of smoke-free workplace legislation on exposures and health: possibilities for prevention. Eur Respir J 2006;28(2):397–408.

54. Schoj V, Alderete M, Ruiz E, et al. The impact of a 100% smoke-free law on the health of hospitality workers from the city of Neuquen, Argentina. Tob Control 2010;19(2):134–7.

55. Massin N, Bohadana AB, Wild P, et al. Respiratory symptoms and bronchial responsiveness in lifeguards exposed to nitrogen trichloride in indoor swimming pools. Occup Environ Med 1998;55(4):258–63.

56. Nemery B, Hoet PH, Nowak D. Indoor swimming pools, water chlorination and respiratory health. Eur Respir J 2002;19(5):790–3.

57. Thickett KM, McCoach JS, Gerber JM, et al. Occupational asthma caused by chloramines in indoor swimming-pool air. Eur Respir J 2002;19(5):827–32.

58. Fantuzzi G, Righi E, Predieri G, et al. Prevalence of ocular, respiratory and cutaneous symptoms in indoor swimming pool workers and exposure to disinfection by-products (DBPs). Int J Environ Res Public Health 2010;7(4):1379–91.

59. Baur X. I are we closer to developing threshold limit values for allergens in the workplace? Ann Allergy Asthma Immunol 2003;90(5 Suppl 2):11–8.

60. Gautrin D, Ghezzo H, Infante-Rivard C, et al. Long-term outcomes in a prospective cohort of apprentices exposed to high-molecular-weight agents. Am J Respir Crit Care Med 2008;177(8):871–9.

61. LaMontagne AD, Radi S, Elder DS, et al. Primary prevention of latex related sensitisation and occupational asthma: a systematic review. Occup Environ Med 2006; 63(5):359–64.

62. Anees W, Moore VC, Burge PS. FEV1 decline in occupational asthma. Thorax 2006;61(9):751–5.

Old and New Causes of Occupational Asthma

Santiago Quirce, MD[a], Jonathan A. Bernstein, MD[b],*

KEYWORDS

- Occupational asthma • Low molecular weight
- High molecular weight • Asthmagens

The earliest account of an occupational asthma (OA) cause was attributed to Hippocrates (460–370 BCE), who described panting, a literal translation of asthma, in metal workers, fullers, tailors, horsemen, farmhands, and fishermen. His perceptive observations have been confirmed in the modern era in that OA has been well characterized in all of these occupations. OA and other respiratory disorders became more widely accepted in the medical community after Bernardino Ramazzini wrote his treatise, "De morbis artificum diatriba" in 1713, which described asthma in bakers; grain handlers; and silk, hemp, and flax workers. OA rapidly accelerated in the twentieth century with the advent of new technologies introducing a spectrum of new agents into the workplace. In the latter half of the twentieth century, the low-molecular-weight (LMW) chemical agents were first recognized as potential respiratory sensitizers that could cause OA. Presently, occupational asthmagens are categorized as LMW (<1000 kd) and high-molecular-weight (HMW, ≥1000 kd) agents. HMW agents are further subclassified as plant or animal derived.

International reviews suggest that the median proportion of adult cases of asthma attributable to occupational exposure is between 10% and 15%.[1] Therefore, it is essential that clinicians have a broad knowledge of the various causes associated with this condition. The purpose of this article is to review the most common representative causes of OA over the past 70 years, with specific emphasis on newer causes that have been reported over the past 5 years.

OLD CAUSES OF OCCUPATIONAL ASTHMA

Traditionally, causes of OA are divided into HMW and LMW agents. These causes have been widely reviewed and most extensively in the text, *Asthma in the Workplace*,

[a] Department Allergy, Hospital La Paz Health Research Institute (IdiPAZ), Madrid, Spain
[b] Division of Immunology/Allergy Section, Department of Internal Medicine, University of Cincinnati College of Medicine, Cincinnati, OH, USA
* Corresponding author. 3255 Eden Avenue, ML#563; Suite 250, Cincinnati, OH 45267-0563.
E-mail address: Jonathan.Bernstein@uc.edu

Immunol Allergy Clin N Am 31 (2011) 677–698
doi:10.1016/j.iac.2011.07.001   immunology.theclinics.com
0889-8561/11/$ – see front matter © 2011 Elsevier Inc. All rights reserved.

published in 1993 and updated in subsequent editions. This text was the first to extensively review the most prevalent causes of OA. The HMW agents that were considered most relevant were flour dusts, enzymes (both plant and animal derived), gums, foods and tobacco, rubber-derived proteins, animal- and insect-derived allergens, and fish/seafood-derived allergens (**Table 1**). The LMW agents considered most relevant were polyisocyanates and their polymers, acid anhydrides, metals, a spectrum of chemical substances (ie, azobisformamide, amines, colophony and fluxes, formaldehyde, persulfate, diazonium salts and reactive dyes, pharmaceuticals, polyvinylchloride and adhesives and acrylates), and western red cedar (see **Table 1**). Irritant-induced asthma, including the reactive airways dysfunction syndrome, is considered a form of OA caused by nonspecific exposure to high levels of irritating vapors, fumes, or smoke and is discussed elsewhere in this monograph. Occupational respiratory disorders, including airway obstruction caused by cotton dusts and organic dust toxic syndrome, are asthmalike conditions but do not fall within the definition of OA. In reviewing the causes of OA over the past 50 to 70 years, it is important to note that many of the reported case series lack confirmatory evidence of OA, including skin testing or specific bronchoprovocation testing (see **Table 1**).

High-Molecular-Weight Agents

In the workplace, HMW protein allergens are natural sensitizers. Baker's asthma, described initially by Thiel and Ulmer[2] in 1980, is a classic example. Subsequently, several studies have reported sensitizing cereal and noncereal grain antigens contained in wheat, triticale, rye, barley, oats, rice, and corn in the workplace.[3] Other relevant allergens associated with baker's asthma include fungal antigens (*Aspergillus* and *Alternaria*); enzymes derived from the *Aspergillus* species, such as α-amylase and hemicellulase; plant-derived enzymes, such as papain/chymopapain; as well as mite antigens.[4–8]

Enzymes are proteins used as biocatalysts to reduce or replace the use of chemicals in a variety of processes.[9] As catalysts, enzymes are used in a variety of industries, including cleaning, food processing, animal feed, fuel alcohol, textile, paper, and pharmaceuticals. The first enzyme commercially introduced in the United States and England was Alcalase in 1967, which was derived from *Bacillus subtilis* for use in soap detergents.[10] Within 3 years, 80% of all soap detergents sold in the United States contained enzymes. Subsequently, Flindt and Pepys[10,11] reported the first cases of respiratory symptoms in detergent workers after inhalation exposure to the *Bacillus subtilis*–derived powdered enzymes, Alcalase and Maxatase. Eighty percent of workers with respiratory symptoms elicited a positive wheal and flare skin test response to skin test reagents prepared from the enzymatic material and *Bacillus subtilis* spore extracts.[10] These index cases demonstrated that enzymes were highly allergenic and that susceptible workers exposed to these agents were at an increased risk for becoming sensitized and developing asthma.

In general, enzymes are plant or microbial derived. Examples of plant-derived enzymes known to cause occupational sensitization and asthma include papain widely used in cosmetic, food, and pharmaceutical consumer products; chymopapain (a proteolytic enzyme, structurally related to papain), once used for intradiscal dissolution of herniated lumbar disks; pepsin used as an additive in the production of liquors, cheeses, and cereals; and bromelain, which is used in the pharmaceutical industry.[9]

Microbial-derived enzymes are typically produced by bacterial microorganisms belonging to *Bacillus* sp and *Pseudomonas* sp and fungal organisms, such as *Aspergillus* sp, *Streptomyces* sp, and *Trichoderma* sp, and are most commonly used to

Table 1
Representative older causes of occupational asthma induced by high-molecular-weight agents

Agents	Occupation	N	Skin Test (%)	Specific IgE	Bronchoprovocation	References
High-Molecular-Weight Agents						
Laboratory animal	Laboratory workers	296	13	34	ND	Venables,[15] 1988
Cow dander	Agricultural workers	49	100	ND	ND	Mantyjarvi, 1992
Egg protein	Egg producers	188	34	29	ND	Smith, 1990
Crab	Snow-crab processors	303	22	ND	72% of 42+	Cartier, 1984
Prawn	Prawn processors	50	26	16	2/2+	Gaddie,[20] 1980
Hoya	Oyster farm	1413	82% of 511+	89% of 180+	ND	Jyo,[25] 1980
Cuttlefish	Deep-sea fishers	66	ND	ND	ND	Tamaszumas, 1988
Salmon	Processing plant	291	ND	25	ND	Douglas,[24] 1995
Red soft coral	Fishers	74	2/2+	ND	ND	Onizuka,[26] 1990
Grain mite	Farmers	290	21	19% of 219+	ND	Cuthbert, 1984
Grain mite	Grain-store workers	133	25	23% of 128+	1/1+	Blainey, 1989
Amblyseius cucumeris (bell pepper pollen)	Horticulturists	472	23	Some	ND	Groenewoud, 2002
Locust	Laboratory workers	118	32% of 113+	Done	ND	Burge, 1980
Screw worm fly	Flight crews	182	91% of 11+	ND	ND	Gibbons, 1965
Insect larvae	Fish-bait handlers	76	32	19	ND	Siracusa, 2003
Fruit fly	Laboratory workers	22	27	27	ND	Spieksma, 1986
Mealworm larvae	Fish-bait handlers	5	4/5	3/5	ND	Bernstein, 1983
Larva of silkworm	Sericulture	5519	100% of 9+	1/1+	100% of 9+	Armentia, 1998
Grain dust	Grain elevators	610	9	ND	ND	Chan-Yeung, 1985
Wheat, rye, and soya flour	Bakers, millers	279	9	ND	ND	Musk et al,[6] 1989
Coffee bean	Food processor	372	24	12	ND	Jones, 1982
Rose	Culture of roses	290	ND	19.5	ND	Demir, 2002

(continued on next page)

Table 1
(continued)

Agents	Occupation	N	Skin Test (%)	Specific IgE	Bronchoprovocation	References
Chrysanthemum	Greenhouse workers	104	20.2	+ in some	ND	Groenewoud, 2002
Helianthus annuus	Processing workers	102	23	ND	ND	Atis, 2002
Biologic enzymes (*Bacillus subtilis*)	Detergent industry	1642	4.5%–75.5%	ND	ND	Juniper, 1977
Papain	Pharmaceutical	29	34	34	89% of 9+	Baur, 1982
Fungal amylase	Bakers	118	100% of 10+	ND	ND	Baur et al,[4] 1986
Fungal amyloglucosidase and hemicellulase	Bakers	140	ND	5%–24%	ND	Baur et al,[8] 1988
Esperase	Detergent industry	667	ND	5%	ND	Zachariae, 1981
Lactase	Pharmaceutical	207	31	ND	ND	Muir, 1997
Guar	Carpet manufacturer	162	8	ND	ND	Malo, 1990
Latex	Glove manufacturing	81	11	ND	ND	Tarlo et al,[30] 1990
Low-Molecular-Weight Agents						
Toluene diisocyanates	Polyurethane, plastics, varnish	112	3	0	45% of 11+	Butcher et al,[35] 1976
Toluene diisocyanates	Polyurethane, plastics, varnish	162	ND	ND	57	Mapp et al,[36] 1988
Diphenylmethane diisocyanate	Foundry	11	ND	27	54.5	Zammit-Tabona et al,[37] 1983
Hexamethylene diisocyanate	Spray painters	20	ND	ND	10+	Vandenplas, 1993
Phthalic anhydride	Plastics	118	18% of 11+	ND	ND	Wenfors, 1986
Trimellitic anhydride	Epoxy resins, plastics	4	100	75	100% of 1+	Zeiss et al,[41] 1977
Aliphatic amines	Chemical factory	12	NA	ND	ND	Ng, 1995
Ethanolamines	Beauty culture	10	ND	ND	100% +	Gelfand, 1963
Quaternary amines	Cleaning product	1	+	ND	+	Bernstein, 1994

Agent	Occupation	N				Reference
Colophony	Electronics workers	34	ND		100%+	Burge, 1980
Western red cedar	Furniture making	1320	19	ND	ND	Ishizaki et al,[44] 1973
Platinum	Platinum refinery	136	17	26	ND	Brooks et al,[48] 1990
Psyllium	Pharmaceutical	130	19% of 120+	26% of 118+	27% of 18+	Bardy et al,[49] 1987
Spiramycin	Pharmaceutical	51	100	ND	25% of 12+	Malo et al,[27] 1988
Reactive dyes	Reactive dyes manufacturer	309	15	34	65% of 20+	Alanko, 1978
Chloramine T	Chemical manufacturing	6	100	ND	ND	Feinberg, 1945
Polyvinyl chloride	Meat wrapper	96	ND	ND	27% of 11+	Andrasch, 1976
Persulfate salts and henna	Hairdressing	23	4	ND	100%	Blainey, 1986
Diazonium salt	Manufacturing of fluorine polymer precursor	45	ND	20	100% of 2	Luczynska, 1990
Azobisformamide	Plastics, rubber	151	ND	ND	ND	Slovak, 1981
Formaldehyde	Hospital staff	28	ND	ND	50% of 4+	Hendrick, 1975
Methyl-methacrylate	Adhesive	7	ND	ND	86%+	Lozewicz et al,[103] 1985

Abbreviations: N, number of workers; ND, not done.
Modified from Malo JL, Chan-Yeung M. Agents causing occupational asthma with key references. In: Bernstein IL, Malo JL, Chan-Yeung M, et al, editors. Asthma in the workplace. 3rd edition. New York: Taylor and Francis; 2006. p. 825–66; with permission.

manufacture soap detergents.[9] These serine protease enzymes derived from *Bacillus* organisms (also called subtilisins or subtilopeptidases) are also useful in household cleaning agents because of their potent enzymatic activity and stability over wide ranges of pH and temperature.[12]

OA induced by cellulose and β-d-galactoside derived from the *Aspergillus niger and oryzae* species, respectively, have been well documented in the pharmaceutical industry.[9] A cross-sectional survey performed on 94 pharmaceutical workers exposed to *Aspergillus oryzae*–derived β-d-galactoside galactohydrolase revealed that 29% of exposed workers had lactase sensitization and lactase-sensitized workers were 9 times more likely to experience upper- or lower-respiratory symptoms compared with skin test negative subjects.[13] Atopic workers were 4 times more likely to develop lactase sensitization compared with nonatopic workers. Reduction of lactase exposure and restricting atopic workers from working with lactase successfully prevented lactase-induced occupational symptoms.[13] Other examples of microbial-derived enzymes causing sensitization and OA include workers exposed to pectinases in the food industry, phytase and β-gluconase in the animal feed industry, and porcine pancreatic amylase in a laboratory.[9]

Egg-processing workers are at an increased risk for OA after becoming sensitized to egg proteins, such as ovalbumin, ovomucoid, and conalbumin, as well as egg lysozyme.[13,14] OA in laboratory animal handlers has been well documented.[15] Atopy is a risk factor for animal handler's OA. Exposed workers typically become sensitized within the first year and the most common cause is rats, followed by mice and rabbits.[16]

Fish and seafood–derived allergens are common causes of OA.[17–26] Many of these workers are fishers or processors that have frequent dermal and inhalational exposure to these allergens.[17–26] Specific immunoglobulin (Ig) E antibody responses have been demonstrated for cuttlefish, trout, shrimp, prawn, crab, and oyster processors and in many instances confirmed by specific bronchoprovocation.[17–27]

OA caused by natural rubber latex sensitization (NRL) was first reported in 1987.[28] Since that time, numerous cross-sectional studies have reported that NRL protein allergens from the rubber tree *Hevea brasiliensis* caused OA in health care workers using high-protein powdered latex gloves, glove manufacturers, and several other occupations.[28–31] Latex-induced OA is an excellent example illustrating the effectiveness of modifying exposure in the workplace in preventing symptoms in workers with established NRL sensitization or OA and in preventing new cases. Since latex-safe environments have been instituted in hospitals by switching to low-protein latex and nonlatex gloves, the prevalence of latex sensitization and reported new cases of OA have dramatically decreased.[32]

Low Molecular Weights

Diisocyanates are LMW chemicals widely used to produce polyurethane foam insulation and spray paints that have wide applications in the automobile and building industries. These chemicals may at times act as haptens and conjugate to endogenous proteins to form complete allergens. Soon after toluene diisocyanate (TDI) was introduced commercially, reports of asthma in exposed workers were reported.[33] Since that time, diisocyantes have become recognized as one of the most common causes of OA in the world. The structural differences between the aromatic compounds, TDI and methylene diphenyl diisocyanate (MDI), and the aliphatic compound, hexamethylene diisocyanate (HDI), confer different chemical properties leading to different exposure risks for workers.[34] For example, TDI is highly volatile at room temperature and is now used less than MDI, which requires heating before vapors are emitted.[34] Many specific bronchoprovocation studies have confirmed that isocyanates are respiratory sensitizers causing OA but specific IgE-mediated sensitization can be demonstrated in only a minority of workers with OA caused by MDI, TDI, or HDI.[31,35–37]

Trimellitic anhydride (TMA) is an acid anhydride widely used as a curing or hardening agent in epoxy resins, in the production of plasticizers for polyvinyl chloride, and in polyester and alkyd resins.[38] The National Institute of Occupational Safety and Health estimates that 20,000 workers in the United States have developed TMA-induced occupational illness in various work processes.[39] TMA can cause irritant-induced asthma after a single large exposure as well as a spectrum of occupational respiratory conditions, asthma being the most common. TMA is a unique LMW chemical because it binds to endogenous protein to form a complete antigen capable of eliciting IgE sensitization that can be demonstrated by skin prick testing or serologically.[40,41] Studies have reported workers becoming sensitized to TMA and have confirmed OA by specific bronchoprovocation.[40,41]

Milne[42,43] first described western red cedar asthma in the timber industry in 1969. Since that time, numerous cases of OA have been described in furniture factory workers, sawmill workers, and other woodworker occupations.[44,45] The constituent thought to induce respiratory sensitization and asthma is plicatic acid.[45]

The most well-described cause of OA induced by metals has been in the platinum refinery industry.[46–48] Exposed workers have been reported to develop positive IgE-specific skin and serologic tests to platinum salts.[46–48] The persistence of sensitization and asthma can be quite prolonged after workers are removed from the workplace, especially if there is a significant delay in removing these workers from further exposure after recognizing the development of sensitization.[48]

Finally, numerous cases of OA have been reported among workers in the pharmaceutical manufacturing industry. Psyllium, which is manufactured as a laxative, has been found to induce IgE sensitization and asthma in susceptible exposed workers.[49] Bardy and colleagues[49] evaluated 130 pharmaceutical workers exposed to psyllium and found that 39 had symptoms suggestive of OA; 23 of 120 workers were skin test positive to psyllium and 31 of 118 workers had specific IgE antibodies to psyllium. Five of 18 workers able to undergo specific bronchoprovocation testing to psyllium were positive.[49]

NEW CAUSES OF OCCUPATIONAL ASTHMA

The high-risk occupations and industries associated with the development of OA vary depending on the predominant industrial sectors in a particular country.[50,51] The list of causative agents of immunologically mediated OA is continuously growing, and new agents and professions are described each year (**Table 2**). A variety of novel HMW and LMW agents have been shown to induce OA. Recent data indicate that LMW chemicals account for more new cases of OA caused by sensitization than HMW agents.[52,53]

HIGH-MOLECULAR-WEIGHT AGENTS
Food and Baking Industry

There are many foods, food additives, and contaminants that have been associated with OA.[54] Exposure to food allergens occurs primarily through inhalation of dust, powder, vapors, and aerosolized proteins generated during cutting, cleaning, cooking or boiling, and drying activities. In the last few years, novel wheat allergens have been implicated in the pathogenesis of baker's asthma. Constantin and colleagues[55] identified in 2008 a serine proteinase inhibitor as a novel allergen in baker's asthma by

Table 2
New causes of occupational asthma

HMW Agents	Occupation	Confirmed By	IgE Pos (+ or -) and to Which Specific Allergens	Reference
Brassica oleracea pollen (cauliflower and broccoli)	Plant breeders	Clinical history	SPT+ IgE+	Hermanides et al,[112] 2006
Korean ginseng & sanyak	Herbal-products trader	SIC+	SPT+ to both IgE+ to sanyak IgE- to ginseng	Lee et al,[113] 2006
Yarrow (*Achillea millefolium*) and Safflower (*Carthamus tinctorious*)	Florist	SIC+	SPT+ IgE+	Compes et al,[114] 2006
Cedrorana (*Cedrelinga catenaeformis* Ducke) wood dust	Carpenter	SIC+	SPT+ IgE+	Eire et al,[72] 2006
Roe deer (*Capreolus capreolus*)	Animal-rehabilitation workers	CPT+	SPT+ IgE+	Carballada et al,[76] 2006
Mushroom (*Pleurotus ostreatus*)	Grocer	SIC+	SPT+ IgE+	Vereda et al,[115] 2007
Arabidopsis thaliana	Laboratory plant worker	SIC+ PEF monitoring	SPT+	Yates et al,[116] 2008
Chamomile (*Matricaria chamomilla*)	Tea-packing-plant worker	SIC+	SPT+ IgE+	Vandenplas et al,[117] 2008
Ivy (*Hedera helix*)	Florist	SIC+ PEF monitoring	SPT-	Hannu et al,[95] 2008
Linseed oilcake (*Linum usitatissimum*)	Chemist	SIC+	SPT+ IgE+	Vandenplas et al,[118] 2008
Tomato (*Lycopersicum esculentum*)	Greenhouse worker	SIC+	SPT+ IgE+	Vandenplas et al,[119] 2008

Tampico fiber (Agave lechuguilla)	Brush maker	SPT+ IgE+	SIC+	Quirce et al,[75] 2008
Olive fruit (Olea europaea)	Olive oil mill worker	SPT+ IgE+ Thaumatinlike protein	NPT+	Palomares et al,[59] 2008
Octopus (Octopus vulgaris)	Seafood processor	SPT+ IgE+	SIC+	Rosado et al,[68] 2009
Bovine serum albumin (Bos d 6)	Laboratory researcher	IgE+	SIC+	Choi et al,[78] 2009
Malt	Machine operator at a malt company	SPT+	SIC+	Miedinger et al,[61] 2009
Chengal wood (Neobalanocarpus hemeii)	Carpenter	ND	SIC+ PEF monitoring	Lee and Tan,[73] 2009
Sausage mold (Penicillium nalgiovensis)	Semi-industrial pork butchers	SPT+	Clinical history	Talleu et al,[82] 2009
Marigold flour (Tagetes erecta)	Animal fodder factory employee	SPT+ IgE+	NPT+	Lluch-Pérez et al,[64] 2009
Cabreuva wood (Myrocarpus frondosus)	Parquet floor layer	SPT- IgE+ BAT+	SIC+	Pala et al,[74] 2010
Rice (Oryza sativa)	Rice mill workers and handlers	SPT+ IgE+	SIC+	Kim et al,[62] 2010
Turbot (Scophthalmus maximus)	Fish-farm workers	SPT+ IgE+	PEF monitoring	Pérez Carral et al,[67] 2010
Gerbil (Meriones unguiculatus)	Biologist	SPT+ IgE+ 23-kDa lipocalin	SIC+	de las Heras et al,[77] 2010
Cellar spider (Holocnemus pluchei)	Farmer	SPT+ IgE+ Arginine kinase	SIC+	Bobolea et al,[85] 2010
LMW agents				

(continued on next page)

Table 2
(continued)

HMW Agents	Occupation	Confirmed By	IgE Pos (+ or -) and to Which Specific Allergens	Reference
Escin	Pharmaceutical worker	SIC+	SPT- IgE-	Munoz et al,[86] 2006
Sevoflurane and isoflurane	Anesthetic staff	SIC+ PEF monitoring	ND	Vellore et al,[87] 2006
Ortho-phthalaldehyde	Nurse	Clinical history	ND	Fujita et al,[88] 2006
Lasamide	Pharmaceutical workers	SIC+	ND	Klusackova et al,[89] 2007
Alendronate	Pharmaceutical worker	SIC+ (occupational rhinitis)	SPT+	Pala et al,[90] 2008
Eugenol	Hairdresser	SIC+	SPT-	Quirce et al,[94] 2008
Turpentine	Art painter	SIC+	SPT-	Dudek et al,[96] 2009
Metal arc welding of iron	Welder	SIC+	ND	Muñoz et al,[97] 2009
Vancomycin	Pharmaceutical worker	PEF monitoring	SPT-, IDT+ IgE- BAT+	Choi et al,[91] 2009
Trimethylolpropane triacrylate	Thermal printer	SIC+	ND	Sánchez-García et al,[111] 2009
Dodecanedioic acid	Electronics instructor	SIC+ PEF monitoring	ND	Moore et al,[98] 2009
Rhodium salts	Operator of an electroplating plant	SIC+	SPT+ IgE-	Merget et al,[99] 2010
5-ASA	Pharmaceutical worker	SIC+	SPT-	Sastre et al,[92] 2010
Colistin	Pharmaceutical worker	SIC+	IgE-	Gómez-Ollés et al,[93] 2010
Polymethyl methacrylate (from eyeglasses)	Optical laboratory technicians	SIC+ PEF monitoring	ND	Quirce et al,[110] 2011

Abbreviations: BAT, basophil activation test; CPT, conjunctival provocation test; IDT, intradermal test; ND, not done; NPT, nasal provocation test; PEF, peak expiratory flow; Pos, positive; SIC, specific inhalation challenge; SPT, skin prick test.

screening of a cDNA library from wheat seeds with serum IgE from patients with asthma. The allergen is a 9.9 kDa protein, which represents a new member of the potato inhibitor I family. It is probably involved in plant defense and belongs to the pathogenesis-related protein-6 family. Palacin and colleagues[56] have characterized wheat Tri a 14 as a major allergen associated with baker's asthma. Specific IgE to this wheat flour was detected in 60% of sera from 40 Spanish patients with baker's asthma, and positive skin prick tests (SPT) were found in 15 (62%) of 24 of these patients. Furthermore, recombinant Tri a 14 has been produced in *Pichia pastoris*; its physicochemical properties, heat and proteolytic resistance, and IgE-binding capacity were shown to be almost equivalent to those of its natural counterpart.[57] Thaumatinlike proteins (TLPs) are the latest salt-soluble protein family from wheat flour that has been associated with baker's respiratory allergy by Lehto and colleagues[58] in 2010. Most TLPs have molecular masses ranging from 21 to 26 kDa. Moreover, OA caused by a TLP from olive fruit has been described.[59] An SPT with purified TLP at 1 µg/ml was positive, as was the nasal challenge test with TLP (0.1 µg/ml).

Constantin and colleagues[60] analyzed the IgE reactivity profiles of patients suffering from baker's asthma, wheat-induced food allergy and grass pollen allergy to microarrayed recombinant wheat flour allergens and grass pollen allergens. They identified recombinant wheat flour allergens, which are specifically recognized by patients suffering from baker's asthma. Profilin was identified as a cross-reactive allergen recognized by patients suffering from baker's asthma and food and pollen allergies.

Miedinger and colleagues[61] reported for the first time a case of IgE-mediated OA to malt in a machine operator for a malt manufacturing company.

Kim and colleagues[62] reported 3 cases of OA caused by exposure to rice powder in the work environment. All 3 patients showed positive SPT and IgE determinations to rice extract, and specific inhalation challenge (SIC) induced immediate and late asthmatic responses.

Pirson and colleagues[63] described the case of a patient working in a factory producing inulin from chicory who developed rhinoconjunctivitis and asthma from the dust of dry chicory roots. An SIC with dry chicory elicited acute rhinoconjunctivitis and an early asthmatic response. SPT results were positive to birch pollen and fresh/dry chicory and negative for inulin. Specific IgE to rBet v 1 was strongly positive. IgE immunoblotting with chicory extract showed a 17 kDa IgE-binding band, which was inhibited with purified Bet v 1.

Marigold flour, prepared from the flowers of *Tagetes erecta* or the flowers of *Calendula officinalis*, has been extensively used by the food additive industry as poultry feed colorant. Lluch-Pérez and colleagues[64] reported the first case of IgE-mediated occupational rhinitis and asthma caused by marigold flour. It was demonstrated by SPT, nasal challenge test, and specific IgE determination. A 60 kDa IgE-binding band was observed by immunoblotting, and cross-reactivity between extracts from marigold flour and *Helianthus annuus* pollen was demonstrated.

Bernstein and colleagues[65] described a case of respiratory sensitization to konjac flour (glucomannan) occurring in a food manufacturing worker. The worker presented with 3 episodes of hives, shortness of breath, chest tightness, wheezing, and hoarseness after exposure to a variety of powdered food ingredients. The evaluation included spirometry, methacholine challenge, and allergy testing to standard allergens and extracts made from food ingredients from the workplace. Serum-specific IgG and IgE enzyme-linked immunosorbent assay (ELISA), ELISA inhibition assays, and specific provocation to relevant food ingredients were also performed. SPT was significantly positive to konjac glucomannan (KGM) and guar gum F glactomannan. Sensitization was confirmed by SIC using a sifting technique. After sifting KGM for 5 minutes, the patient developed upper- and lower-respiratory symptoms associated with a significant decrease in peak expiratory flow rate requiring emergency treatment. Subsequent avoidance of KGM in the workplace resulted in the resolution of all symptoms. This case demonstrates the potentially sensitizing nature of polysaccharide-based food additives that can lead to severe allergic reactions.[65]

Lucas and colleagues[66] have reviewed OA in the commercial fishing industry, indicating that it more commonly occurs because of crustaceans, but mollusks and finfish are also implicated. Pérez Carral and colleagues[67] reported 3 workers at a fish farm who experienced rhinoconjunctivitis and asthma caused by sensitization to turbot. The allergens were parvalbumin in 1 case and a different allergen in the remaining 2 patients.

Rosado and colleagues[68] described the first case of OA from aerosolized octopus allergens in a seafood-processing worker. Immunoblotting revealed IgE-binding bands of 43 and 32 kDa that could correspond to tropomyosin.

OA caused by exposure to the fish and nematode parasite, *Anisakis simplex*, through an IgE-mediated mechanism has also been reported among fish processors.[69]

Wood and Vegetal Fiber

Wood-dust exposure may cause IgE-mediated allergic diseases. Schlünssen and colleagues[70] reported that the prevalence of pine and beech sensitization among current Danish woodworkers was 1.7% and 3.1%, respectively. No differences in sensitization rates were found between woodworkers and references, but the prevalence of wood-dust sensitization was dose-dependently associated to the current level of wood-dust exposure. They suggested that the importance of beech and pine-wood sensitization may be of clinical significance for a few workers if the IgE epitopes are proteinaceous.

Campo and colleagues[71] evaluated the frequency of work-related specific sensitization and respiratory symptoms in carpentry apprentices with exposure to wood dust and diisocyanates. SPTs to a panel of 14 different woods were performed in 101 apprentices. Sensitization to wood was detected in 9% of the participants, all of whom were atopic with a history of rhinitis; 2 of them had asthma. Seven apprentices showed a positive SPT reaction to olive tree wood, 1 to obeche wood, and 1 to pine tree wood.

Eire and colleagues[72] described a carpenter who developed occupational rhinitis and asthma caused by cedrorana (*Cedrelinga catenaeformis Ducke*) wood dust. SPT and specific IgE to this wood were positive. Both nasal provocation and SIC to cedrorana wood elicited early responses.[72]

Chengal is a resistant rainforest hardwood that is commonly used in Southeast Asia. Exposure to chengal wood dust can lead to OA and rhinitis of an uncertain mechanism.[73]

Pala and colleagues[74] reported the case of an atopic man employed as a parquet floor layer who developed occupational rhinitis and asthma caused by cabreuva wood (*Myrocarpus frondosus*). SPT with cabreuva wood dust was negative, and SIC elicited rhinitis and a dual asthmatic response. IgE reactivity toward a 75-kDa protein and a positive basophil activation test strongly suggested a role of IgE in cabreuva wood–induced respiratory allergy.

Two brush-making workers who developed asthma and rhinitis symptoms following occupational exposure to Tampico fiber were described.[75] Tampico fiber, which is extracted from the leaves of *Agave lechuguilla*, is used extensively for making yard brooms, deck brushes, and bath brushes. SPTs and IgE-immunoblotting to Tampico extract were positive. The results of SIC and induced sputum supported an effect of Tampico fiber exposure in causing OA on a nonirritating basis.[75]

Animal and Arthropod Allergens

Occupational rhinitis and asthma caused by roe deer-derived allergens has been described in two workers at an animal rehabilitation center.[76] De las Heras and colleagues[77] have described a biologist who developed rhinitis and OA when she worked with gerbils (*Meriones unguiculatus*). A new gerbil allergen of 23 kDa was identified in the gerbil urine, epithelium, hair, and airborne samples. Partial characterization of this allergen suggested that it was possibly a lipocalin.

Bos d 6, bovine serum albumin (BSA), is a major allergen in beef and a minor allergen in milk. It is also commonly used in research laboratories. Choi and colleagues[78] reported a case of OA and rhinitis in a laboratory worker caused by the inhalation of BSA powder in which an IgE-mediated response was demonstrated.

OA caused by the mold *Chrysonilia sitophila* (asexual state of *Neurospora sitophila*), which was previously reported in the lodging industry, has been recently shown to also affect workers in the coffee industry. OA has been demonstrated by SPT, serial peak expiratory flow (PEF) measurements, and IgE analyses.[79–81]

A case of chronic cough related to OA with sensitivity to dry sausage mold (*Penicillium nalgiovensis*) has been reported in a semi-industrial pork butcher worker.[82] The diagnosis was based on positive SPT, spirometry, and a favorable outcome after avoidance of the allergen.

Miedinger and colleagues[83] have described the case of an engineer who worked for an electric power company who developed OA caused by caddis flies (Phryganeiae) confirmed by a SIC using an extract of these insects.

Amblyseius californicus has been recently added to the list of predatory mites that induced IgE sensitization and OA among greenhouse workers.[84]

Bobolea and colleagues[85] have recently reported a case of OA in a farmer caused by the cellar spider (*Holocnemus pluchei*) and confirmed by SIC. Immunoblotting displayed different bands in the spider extract, in a range of 20 to 70 kDa. All were hemocyanins, except for a 17-kDa protein identified as an arginine kinase.

LOW-MOLECULAR-WEIGHT AGENTS
Escin

A 57-year-old man employed in the pharmaceutical industry developed asthma while working with *Plantago ovata* and escin, an active ingredient derived from horse chestnut with antiinflammatory and venotonic properties. An SIC with escin was positive, whereas SIC with *P ovata* was negative. The mechanism by which escin can produce asthma is unknown, but possibly non-IgE mediated.[86]

Sevoflurane and Isoflurane

Three cases of OA, work-related angioedema or dermatitis to isoflurane (1-chloro-2,2,2-trifluoroethyl difluoromethyl ether) and sevoflurane (fluoromethyl 2,2,2-trifluoro-1-[trifluoromethyl] ethyl ether), were described in anesthetic assistants or nurses in the same hospital. All presented a positive SIC. In 2 patients, a late asthmatic response was elicited after SIC (one with isoflurane and sevoflurane and another with sevoflurane). In another patient, exposure to isoflurane was followed by an itchy rash.[87]

Ortho-phthalaldehyde

A nurse employed in the endoscopic unit developed asthma and contact dermatitis a few months after starting to work with ortho-phthalaldehyde for the disinfection of endoscopes.[88]

Lasamide

Lasamide (2,4-dichloro-5-sulfamoylbenzoic acid) is used in the manufacture of the diuretic furosemide (4-chloro-N-furfuryl-5-sulfamoylanthranilic acid). Three patients from a lasamide production line were diagnosed with OA. All 3 patients had positive SIC. Two patients were diagnosed with occupational rhinitis.[89]

Alendronate

Sodium alendronate (SA) is an LMW compound inhibiting bone resorption that is used to treat osteoporosis. A woman employed in a pharmaceutical company started to complain of nasal itching, rhinorrhea, and dry cough 1 month after being moved exclusively to the SA line. SPT and patch tests with SA in saline were positive. An SIC with exposure for 60 minutes to SA 10 mg dissolved in lactose provoked a significant increase in the nasal symptoms score and a significant decrease in peak nasal inspiratory flow but no change in FEV_1. After SA exposure, bronchial hyperresponsiveness to methacholine and induced sputum eosinophils increased.[90]

Vancomycin

A 33-year-old man, employed in the pharmaceutical industry, developed rhinorrhea, cough, dyspnea, and chest discomfort at work, which consisted of purifying vancomycin to manufacture into its powder form. The diagnosis of vancomycin-induced OA was based on clinical history, work-related symptoms, and increased PEF variability at the workplace.[91]

5-Aminosalicylic Acid

A 56-year-old man complained of cough, dyspnea, and wheezing 1 month after beginning work in manufacturing a drug containing 5-aminosalicylic acid (5-ASA), despite taking measures to protect the skin and respiratory system. SPT to 5-ASA (10 mg/mL) was negative. PC_{20} methacholine was greater than 16 mg/mL, fractionated exhaled nitric oxide (FENO) level was 32 ppb, and induced sputum showed no eosinophils. During an SIC, the patient was exposed to 5-ASA (5% in lactose) in the chamber at a mean concentration of 2.65 mg/m^3 for a total of 30 minutes. A late response was observed 9 hours after the challenge; 24 hours later, methacholine PC_{20} was 10 mg/mL, with a FENO value of 53 ppb and induced sputum showed 65% eosinophils.[92]

Colistin

An atopic 24-year-old man working in a pharmaceutical company transporting and storing raw material developed occupational rhinitis and asthma to colistin. Three months after starting his current job, he developed rhinitis, which improved over the weekends. Nine months after the onset of rhinitis, exposure to colistin caused him to suffer sudden cough, wheeze, and dyspnea. The SIC confirmed the diagnosis of OA and rhinitis to colistin. Specific IgE was not detected.[93]

Eugenol

A hairdresser developed occupational rhinitis and asthma caused by eugenol, confirmed with an SIC test (late asthmatic reaction). SPT with common aeroallergens, latex and eugenol 2% weight per volume, were negative, as well as a patch test with eugenol.[94] An increase in sputum eosinophils and lymphocytes was observed 24 hours after eugenol SIC, and a methacholine inhalation test became positive. Proliferation tests of peripheral blood mononuclear cells from the patient showed a strikingly (15 times higher) different eugenol-induced proliferation as compared with the control subject.[94]

Ivy

A 40-year-old woman who had worked in her own flower shop for the past 11 years developed cough and dyspnea when she handled ivy. SPT with different plants, including *Hedera helix* (leaf), were negative. An SIC during which the patient cut and tore the flowers, stalks, and leaves of the plants for 30 minutes elicited an immediate asthmatic reaction.[95]

Turpentine

Turpentine, a fluid obtained by distillation of wood resins containing a mixture of terpenes, is a known inducer of contact dermatitis. A 27-year-old art painter using turpentine as a thinner for oil-based paints developed asthmatic reactions after 5 years of working with turpentine. An SIC showed a late asthmatic reaction and an increase of eosinophils in sputum 24 hours after the challenge.[96]

Iron Welding Fumes

Muñoz and colleagues[97] described 3 patients with OA secondary to exposure to welding fumes generated during metal arc welding of iron. The exposure time ranged from 7 to 43 years and the time of the onset of symptoms following the start of exposure was 2 to 12 years. Patients were diagnosed by SIC.

Dodecanedioic Acid

Moore and colleagues[98] reported the first case of OA caused by electronic colophony-free gel flux predominantly containing dodecanedioic acid. The patient worked as an electronics instructor, and OA was demonstrated by serial PEF measurements and by a positive SIC with dodecanedioic acid fluxes, whereas the SIC was negative to the colophony wire and wire containing predominantly palmitic acid.

Rhodium Salts

A 27-year-old atopic operator of an electroplating plant developed work-related shortness of breath and runny nose with sneezing after exposure to rhodium salts. The patient showed positive SPT reactions and positive bronchial immediate-type reactions with rhodium and platinum salts.[99]

Triglycidyl Isocyanate

Triglycidyl isocyanate (TGIC) is a hardening agent used in powder paints. TGIC has been reported to cause allergic contact dermatitis, OA, and hypersensitivity pneumonitis in powder paint sprayers.[100] A 28-year-old woman developed work-related asthma symptoms when aluminum frames were treated with an electrostatic powder paint containing 2.5% to 10.0% TGIC.[101] OA was confirmed by serial PEF measurements and a methacholine test. An SIC with TGIC (4% in lactose) at a mean concentration of 3.61 mg/m^3 for 15 minutes induced an isolated early asthmatic response. No IgE to TGIC was detected by ELISA testing and no IgE-binding bands were found by immunoblot analysis. Anees and colleagues[102] reported 6 workers at a factory that made domestic gas appliances that had a powder coat containing 10% TGIC applied to them electrostatically to provide a protective and decorative finish. These workers, who were exposed as bystanders to heated TGIC, developed OA confirmed by serial PEF measurements. SIC testing resulted in late or dual asthmatic reactions to heated TGIC in 4 of the 4 tested and was negative in 3 control subjects with asthma. One worker tested only with unheated TGIC had a negative SIC test. Thus, heated TGIC can cause OA from bystander exposure.

Acrylates

Acrylates are well-known causative agents of occupational rhinitis and asthma.[103,104] The widest series of OA caused by acrylates were reported by Savonius and colleagues and Piirilä and colleagues.[105,106] Jaakkola and colleagues[107] reported that the risk of adult-onset asthma, nasal symptoms, and other respiratory symptoms significantly increases with the daily use of methacrylates in dental assistants' work. Sauni and colleagues[108] recently described the first 2 cases of OA caused by sculptured nails containing methacrylates. Both patients had a dual type of asthmatic reaction after a work simulation test, and 1 of them also had allergic contact dermatitis from exposure to methacrylates. Similarly, Jurado-Palomo and colleagues[109] reported a case of OA caused by cyanoacrylates contained in sculptured fingernails, confirmed by means of SIC, significant changes in airway hyperresponsiveness to methacholine, and an increase in FENO. Quirce and colleagues[110] have recently reported 2 cases of optical laboratory technicians with work-related rhinitis and asthma. Acrylates contained in eyeglass lenses have not been previously reported as an etiological agent of OA. Her job consisted of cutting and polishing eyeglasses made of polycarbonate and polymethyl methacrylate. Sánchez-García and colleagues[111] described a nonatopic, nonsmoking 62-year-old woman who had been working for 20 years selling lottery tickets inside a 4-m^3 kiosk. Over the last 3 years, she had been using a point-of-sale (POS) terminal to print lottery coupons. POS are devices used worldwide to pay with credit cards or to print lottery/bet coupons. She had a 2.5-year history of rhinoconjunctivitis, facial edema, cough, shortness of breath, and wheezing within 30 to 60 minutes after arriving at her workplace, which improved during holidays. SIC in a 7-m^3 chamber in a worker performing painting on a cardboard with the tint provided by the lotto company (containing trimethylolpropane-triacrylate) elicited an early asthmatic reaction. Twenty-four hours after the challenge, methacholine PC_{20} was 1.68 mg/mL (baseline methacholine PC_{20} was 6.18 mg/mL) and FeNO 22 ppb (baseline 14 ppb). Induced sputum cell count showed a 100% increase in eosinophils in comparison with baseline counts. One week later, an occupational-type challenge was performed simulating her work environment using the patient's own POS and printing coupons for 90 seconds, and again an early asthmatic reaction was observed.

REFERENCES

1. Balmes J, Becklake M, Blanc P, et al. American Thoracic Society statement: occupational contribution to the burden of airway disease. Am J Respir Crit Care Med 2003;167(5):787–97.
2. Thiel H, Ulmer WT. Bakers' asthma: development and possibility for treatment. Chest 1980;78(Suppl 2):400–5.
3. Block G, Tse KS, Kijek K, et al. Baker's asthma. Studies of the cross-antigenicity between different cereal grains. Clin Allergy 1984;14(2):177–85.
4. Baur X, Fruhmann G, Haug B, et al. Role of Aspergillus amylase in baker's asthma. Lancet 1986;1(8471):43.

5. Klaustermeyer WB, Bardana EJ Jr, Hale FC. Pulmonary hypersensitivity to Alternaria and Aspergillus in baker's asthma. Clin Allergy 1977;7(3):227–33.
6. Musk AW, Venables KM, Crook B, et al. Respiratory symptoms, lung function, and sensitisation to flour in a British bakery. Br J Ind Med 1989;46(9):636–42.
7. Tarlo SM, Shaikh W, Bell B, et al. Papain-induced allergic reactions. Clin Allergy 1978;8(3):207–15.
8. Baur X, Sauer W, Weiss W. Baking additives as new allergens in baker's asthma. Respiration 1988;54(1):70–2.
9. Bernstein JA, Sarlo K. Enzymes. In: Bernstein IL, Chan-Yeung M, Malo JL, et al, editors. Asthma in the workplace. 3rd edition. Rome (Italy): Taylor and Francis, Inc; 2006. p. 377–92.
10. Flindt ML. Pulmonary disease due to inhalation of derivatives of Bacillus subtilis containing proteolytic enzyme. Lancet 1969;1(7607):1177–81.
11. Pepys J, Longbottom JL, Hargreave FE, et al. Allergic reactions of the lungs to enzymes of Bacillus subtilis. Lancet 1969;1(7607):1181–4.
12. Mitchell CA, Gandevia B. Respiratory symptoms and skin reactivity in workers exposed to proteolytic enzymes in the detergent industry. Am Rev Respir Dis 1971;104(1):1–12.
13. Bernstein JA, Bernstein DI, Stauder T, et al. A cross-sectional survey of sensitization to Aspergillus oryzae-derived lactase in pharmaceutical workers. J Allergy Clin Immunol 1999;103(6):1153–7.
14. Bernstein JA, Kraut A, Bernstein DI, et al. Occupational asthma induced by inhaled egg lysozyme. Chest 1993;103(2):532–5.
15. Venables KM, Tee RD, Hawkins ER, et al. Laboratory animal allergy in a pharmaceutical company. Br J Ind Med 1988;45(10):660–6.
16. Davies GE, Thompson AV, Niewola Z, et al. Allergy to laboratory animals: a retrospective and a prospective study. Br J Ind Med 1983;40(4):442–9.
17. Beltrami V, Innocenti A, Pieroni MG, et al. [Occupational asthma caused by inhalation of cuttlefish bone dust]. Med Lav 1989;80(5):425–8 [in Italian].
18. Carino M, Elia G, Molinini R, et al. Shrimp-meal asthma in the aquaculture industry. Med Lav 1985;76(6):471–5.
19. Cartier A, Malo JL, Ghezzo H, et al. IgE sensitization in snow crab-processing workers. J Allergy Clin Immunol 1986;78(2):344–8.
20. Gaddie J, Legge JS, Friend JA, et al. Pulmonary hypersensitivity in prawn workers. Lancet 1980;2(8208–8209):1350–3.
21. Orford RR, Wilson JT. Epidemiologic and immunologic studies in processors of the king crab. Am J Ind Med 1985;7(2):155–69.
22. Sherson D, Hansen I, Sigsgaard T. Occupationally related respiratory symptoms in trout-processing workers. Allergy 1989;44(5):336–41.
23. Tomaszunas S, Weclawik Z, Lewinski M. Allergic reactions to cuttlefish in deep-sea fishermen. Lancet 1988;1(8594):1116–7.
24. Douglas JD, McSharry C, Blaikie L, et al. Occupational asthma caused by automated salmon processing. Lancet 1995;346(8977):737–40.
25. Jyo T, Kohmoto K, Katsutani T, et al. Hoya (sea-squirt) asthma. In: Frazier CA, editor. Occupational Asthma. London: Von Nostrand Reinhold; 1980. p. 209–28.
26. Onizuka R, Inoue K, Kamiya H. [Red soft coral-induced allergic symptoms observed in spiny lobster fishermen]. Arerugi 1990;39(3):339–47 [in Japanese].
27. Malo JL, Cartier A, Ghezzo H, et al. Patterns of improvement in spirometry, bronchial hyperresponsiveness, and specific IgE antibody levels after cessation of exposure in occupational asthma caused by snow-crab processing. Am Rev Respir Dis 1988;138(4):807–12.

28. Seifert HU, Seifert B, Wahl R, et al. [Immunoglobulin E-mediated contact urticaria and bronchial asthma caused by household rubber gloves containing latex. 3 case reports]. Derm Beruf Umwelt 1987;35(4):137–9 [in German].

29. Bernstein DI. Allergic reactions to workplace allergens. JAMA 1997;278(22): 1907–13.

30. Tarlo SM, Wong L, Roos J, et al. Occupational asthma caused by latex in a surgical glove manufacturing plant. J Allergy Clin Immunol 1990;85(3):626–31.

31. Vandenplas O, Delwiche JP, Evrard G, et al. Prevalence of occupational asthma due to latex among hospital personnel. Am J Respir Crit Care Med 1995;151(1): 54–60.

32. Vandenplas O, Larbanois A, Vanassche F, et al. Latex-induced occupational asthma: time trend in incidence and relationship with hospital glove policies. Allergy 2009;64(3):415–20.

33. Fuchs S, Valade P. Clinical and experimental study of some cases of poisoning by Desmodur T (1-2-4 and 1-2-6 di-isocyanates of toluene). Arch Mal Prof 1951; 12(2):191–6.

34. Seguin P, Allard A, Cartier A, et al. Prevalence of occupational asthma in spray painters exposed to several types of isocyanates, including polymethylene polyphenylisocyanate. J Occup Med 1987;29(4):340–4.

35. Butcher BT, Salvaggio JE, Weill H, et al. Toluene diisocyanate (TDI) pulmonary disease: immunologic and inhalation challenge studies. J Allergy Clin Immunol 1976;58(1 PT 1):89–100.

36. Mapp CE, Boschetto P, Dal Vecchio L, et al. Occupational asthma due to isocyanates. Eur Respir J 1988;1(3):273–9.

37. Zammit-Tabona M, Sherkin M, Kijek K, et al. Asthma caused by diphenylmethane diisocyanate in foundry workers. Clinical, bronchial provocation, and immunologic studies. Am Rev Respir Dis 1983;128(2):226–30.

38. Grammer LC, Shaughnessy MA, Zeiss CR, et al. Review of trimellitic anhydride (TMA) induced respiratory response. Allergy Asthma Proc 1997;18(4):235–7.

39. Available at: http://www.cdc.gov/NIOSH/78121_21.html. 1997. Accessed February 4, 2011.

40. Zeiss CR, Mitchell JH, Van Peenen PF, et al. A clinical and immunologic study of employees in a facility manufacturing trimellitic anhydride. Allergy Proc 1992; 13(4):193–8.

41. Zeiss CR, Patterson R, Pruzansky JJ, et al. Trimellitic anhydride-induced airway syndromes: clinical and immunologic studies. J Allergy Clin Immunol 1977; 60(2):96–103.

42. Gandevia B, Milne J. Occupational asthma and rhinitis due to western red cedar (Thuja plicata), with special reference to bronchial reactivity. Br J Ind Med 1970; 27(3):235–44.

43. Milne J, Gandevia B. Occupational asthma and rhinitis due to western (Canadian) red cedar (Thuja plicata). Med J Aust 1969;2(15):741–4.

44. Ishizaki T, Shida T, Miyamoto T, et al. Occupational asthma from western red cedar dust (Thuja plicata) in furniture factory workers. J Occup Med 1973; 15(7):580–5.

45. Vedal S, Enarson DA, Chan H, et al. A longitudinal study of the occurrence of bronchial hyperresponsiveness in western red cedar workers. Am Rev Respir Dis 1988;137(3):651–5.

46. Baker DB, Gann PH, Brooks SM, et al. Cross-sectional study of platinum salts sensitization among precious metals refinery workers. Am J Ind Med 1990; 18(6):653–64.

47. Biagini RE, Bernstein IL, Gallagher JS, et al. The diversity of reaginic immune responses to platinum and palladium metallic salts. J Allergy Clin Immunol 1985;76(6):794–802.
48. Brooks SM, Baker DB, Gann PH, et al. Cold air challenge and platinum skin reactivity in platinum refinery workers. Bronchial reactivity precedes skin prick response. Chest 1990;97(6):1401–7.
49. Bardy JD, Malo JL, Seguin P, et al. Occupational asthma and IgE sensitization in a pharmaceutical company processing psyllium. Am Rev Respir Dis 1987; 135(5):1033–8.
50. Jeebhay MF, Quirce S. Occupational asthma in the developing and industrialised world: a review. Int J Tuberc Lung Dis 2007;11(2):122–33.
51. Kogevinas M, Zock JP, Jarvis D, et al. Exposure to substances in the workplace and new-onset asthma: an international prospective population-based study (ECRHS-II). Lancet 2007;370(9584):336–41.
52. Maestrelli P, Fabbri LM, Mapp CE. Pathophysiology. In: Bernstein IL, Chang-Yeung M, Malo JL, et al, editors. Asthma in the workplace and related conditions. 3rd edition. New York: Taylor and Francis; 2006. p. 109–40.
53. Sastre J, Vandenplas O, Park HS. Pathogenesis of occupational asthma. Eur Respir J 2003;22(2):364–73.
54. Cartier A. The role of inhalant food allergens in occupational asthma. Curr Allergy Asthma Rep 2010;10(5):349–56.
55. Constantin C, Quirce S, Grote M, et al. Molecular and immunological characterization of a wheat serine proteinase inhibitor as a novel allergen in baker's asthma. J Immunol 2008;180(11):7451–60.
56. Palacin A, Varela J, Quirce S, et al. Recombinant lipid transfer protein Tri a 14: a novel heat and proteolytic resistant tool for the diagnosis of baker's asthma. Clin Exp Allergy 2009;39(8):1267–76.
57. Tordesillas L, Pacios LF, Palacin A, et al. Molecular basis of allergen cross-reactivity: non-specific lipid transfer proteins from wheat flour and peach fruit as models. Mol Immunol 2009;47(2–3):534–40.
58. Lehto M, Airaksinen L, Puustinen A, et al. Thaumatin-like protein and baker's respiratory allergy. Ann Allergy Asthma Immunol 2010;104(2):139–46.
59. Palomares O, Alcantara M, Quiralte J, et al. Airway disease and thaumatin-like protein in an olive-oil mill worker. N Engl J Med 2008;358(12):1306–8.
60. Constantin C, Quirce S, Poorafshar M, et al. Micro-arrayed wheat seed and grass pollen allergens for component-resolved diagnosis. Allergy 2009;64(7): 1030–7.
61. Miedinger D, Malo JL, Cartier A, et al. Malt can cause both occupational asthma and allergic alveolitis. Allergy 2009;64(8):1228–9.
62. Kim JH, Choi GS, Kim JE, et al. Three cases of rice-induced occupational asthma. Ann Allergy Asthma Immunol 2010;104(4):353–4.
63. Pirson F, Detry B, Pilette C. Occupational rhinoconjunctivitis and asthma caused by chicory and oral allergy syndrome associated with bet v 1-related protein. J Investig Allergol Clin Immunol 2009;19(4):306–10.
64. Lluch-Perez M, Garcia-Rodriguez RM, Malet A, et al. Occupational allergy caused by marigold (Tagetes erecta) flour inhalation. Allergy 2009;64(7):1100–1.
65. Bernstein JA, Crandall MS, Floyd R. Respiratory sensitization of a food manufacturing worker to konjac glucomannan. J Asthma 2007;44(8):675–80.
66. Lucas D, Lucas R, Boniface K, et al. Occupational asthma in the commercial fishing industry: a case series and review of the literature. Int Marit Health 2010;61(1):13–6.

67. Perez Carral C, Martin-Lazaro J, Ledesma A, et al. Occupational asthma caused by turbot allergy in 3 fish-farm workers. J Investig Allergol Clin Immunol 2010; 20(4):349–51.

68. Rosado A, Tejedor MA, Benito C, et al. Occupational asthma caused by octopus particles. Allergy 2009;64(7):1101–2.

69. Barbuzza O, Guarneri F, Galtieri G, et al. Protein contact dermatitis and allergic asthma caused by Anisakis simplex. Contact Dermatitis 2009;60(4): 239–40.

70. Schlunssen V, Kespohl S, Jacobsen G, et al. Immunoglobulin E-mediated sensitization to pine and beech dust in relation to wood dust exposure levels and respiratory symptoms in the furniture industry. Scand J Work Environ Health 2011;37(2):159–67.

71. Campo P, Aranda A, Rondon C, et al. Work-related sensitization and respiratory symptoms in carpentry apprentices exposed to wood dust and diisocyanates. Ann Allergy Asthma Immunol 2010;105(1):24–30.

72. Eire MA, Pineda F, Losada SV, et al. Occupational rhinitis and asthma due to cedroarana (Cedrelinga catenaeformis Ducke) wood dust allergy. J Investig Allergol Clin Immunol 2006;16(6):385–7.

73. Lee LT, Tan KL. Occupational asthma due to exposure to chengal wood dust. Occup Med (Lond) 2009;59(5):357–9.

74. Pala G, Pignatti P, Perfetti L, et al. Occupational rhinitis and asthma due to cabreuva wood dust. Ann Allergy Asthma Immunol 2010;104(3):268–9.

75. Quirce S, Fernandez-Nieto M, Pastor C, et al. Occupational asthma due to tampico fiber from agave leaves. Allergy 2008;63(7):943–5.

76. Carballada F, Sanchez R, Carballas C, et al. Occupational respiratory allergy to roe deer. Ann Allergy Asthma Immunol 2006;97(5):707–10.

77. de las Heras M, Cuesta-Herranz J, Cases B, et al. Occupational asthma caused by gerbil: purification and partial characterization of a new gerbil allergen. Ann Allergy Asthma Immunol 2010;104(6):540–2.

78. Choi GS, Kim JH, Lee HN, et al. Occupational asthma caused by inhalation of bovine serum albumin powder. Allergy Asthma Immunol Res 2009;1(1):45–7.

79. Francuz B, Yera H, Geraut L, et al. Occupational asthma induced by Chrysonilia sitophila in a worker exposed to coffee grounds. Clin Vaccine Immunol 2010; 17(10):1645–6.

80. Heffler E, Nebiolo F, Pizzimenti S, et al. Occupational asthma caused by Neurospora sitophila sensitization in a coffee dispenser service operator. Ann Allergy Asthma Immunol 2009;102(2):168–9.

81. Monzon S, Gil J, Ledesma A, et al. Occupational asthma IgE mediated due to Chrysonilia sitophila in coffee industry. Allergy 2009;64(11):1686–7.

82. Talleu C, Delourme J, Dumas C, et al. [Allergic asthma due to sausage mould]. Rev Mal Respir 2009;26(5):557–9 [in French].

83. Miedinger D, Cartier A, Lehrer SB, et al. Occupational asthma to caddis flies (Phryganeiae). Occup Environ Med 2010;67(7):503.

84. Skousgaard SG, Thisling T, Bindslev-Jensen C, et al. Occupational asthma caused by the predatory beneficial mites Amblyseius californicus and Amblyseius cucumeris. Occup Environ Med 2010;67(4):287.

85. Bobolea I, Barranco P, Pastor-Vargas C, et al. Arginine kinase from the cellar spider (Holocnemus pluchei): a new asthma-causing allergen. Int Arch Allergy Immunol 2011;155(2):180–6.

86. Munoz X, Culebras M, Cruz MJ, et al. Occupational asthma related to aescin inhalation. Ann Allergy Asthma Immunol 2006;96(3):494–6.

87. Vellore AD, Drought VJ, Sherwood-Jones D, et al. Occupational asthma and allergy to sevoflurane and isoflurane in anaesthetic staff. Allergy 2006;61(12):1485–6.

88. Fujita H, Ogawa M, Endo Y. A case of occupational bronchial asthma and contact dermatitis caused by ortho-phthalaldehyde exposure in a medical worker. J Occup Health 2006;48(6):413–6.

89. Klusackova P, Lebedova J, Pelclova D, et al. Occupational asthma and rhinitis in workers from a lasamide production line. Scand J Work Environ Health 2007; 33(1):74–8.

90. Pala G, Perfetti L, Cappelli I, et al. Occupational rhinitis to sodium alendronate. Allergy 2008;63(8):1092–3.

91. Choi GS, Sung JM, Lee JW, et al. A case of occupational asthma caused by inhalation of vancomycin powder. Allergy 2009;64(9):1391–2.

92. Sastre J, Garcia del Potro M, Aguado E, et al. Occupational asthma due to 5-aminosalicylic acid. Occup Environ Med 2010;67(11):798–9.

93. Gomez-Olles S, Madrid-San Martin F, Cruz MJ, et al. Occupational asthma due to colistin in a pharmaceutical worker. Chest 2010;137(5):1200–2.

94. Quirce S, Fernandez-Nieto M, del Pozo V, et al. Occupational asthma and rhinitis caused by eugenol in a hairdresser. Allergy 2008;63(1):137–8.

95. Hannu T, Kauppi P, Tuppurainen M, et al. Occupational asthma to ivy (Hedera helix). Allergy 2008;63(4):482–3.

96. Dudek W, Wittczak T, Swierczynska-Machura D, et al. Occupational asthma due to turpentine in art painter–case report. Int J Occup Med Environ Health 2009; 22(3):293–5.

97. Munoz X, Cruz MJ, Freixa A, et al. Occupational asthma caused by metal arc welding of iron. Respiration 2009;78(4):455–9.

98. Moore VC, Manney S, Vellore AD, et al. Occupational asthma to gel flux containing dodecanedioic acid. Allergy 2009;64(7):1099–100.

99. Merget R, Sander I, van Kampen V, et al. Occupational immediate-type asthma and rhinitis due to rhodium salts. Am J Ind Med 2010;53(1):42–6.

100. Quirce S, Fernandez-Nieto M, Gorgolas M, et al. Hypersensitivity pneumonitis caused by triglycidyl isocyanurate. Allergy 2004;59(10):1128.

101. Sastre J, Carnes J, Potro MG, et al. Occupational asthma caused by triglycidyl isocyanurate. Int Arch Occup Environ Health 2011;84(5):547–9.

102. Anees W, Moore VC, Croft JS, et al. Occupational asthma caused by heated triglycidyl isocyanurate. Occup Med (Lond) 2011;61(1):65–7.

103. Lozewicz S, Davison AG, Hopkirk A, et al. Occupational asthma due to methyl methacrylate and cyanoacrylates. Thorax 1985;40(11):836–9.

104. Quirce S, Baeza ML, Tornero P, et al. Occupational asthma caused by exposure to cyanoacrylate. Allergy 2001;56(5):446–9.

105. Piirila P, Kanerva L, Keskinen H, et al. Occupational respiratory hypersensitivity caused by preparations containing acrylates in dental personnel. Clin Exp Allergy 1998;28(11):1404–11.

106. Savonius B, Keskinen H, Tuppurainen M, et al. Occupational respiratory disease caused by acrylates. Clin Exp Allergy 1993;23(5):416–24.

107. Jaakkola MS, Leino T, Tammilehto L, et al. Respiratory effects of exposure to methacrylates among dental assistants. Allergy 2007;62(6):648–54.

108. Sauni R, Kauppi P, Alanko K, et al. Occupational asthma caused by sculptured nails containing methacrylates. Am J Ind Med 2008;51(12):968–74.

109. Jurado-Palomo J, Caballero T, Fernandez-Nieto M, et al. Occupational asthma caused by artificial cyanoacrylate fingernails. Ann Allergy Asthma Immunol 2009;102(5):440–1.

110. Quirce S, Barranco P, Fernández-Nieto M, et al. Occupational asthma caused by acrylates in optical laboratory technicians. J Investig Allergol Clin Immunol 2011;21(1):78–9.

111. Sanchez-Garcia S, Fernandez-Nieto M, Sastre J. Asthma induced by a thermal printer. N Engl J Med 2009;360(22):2375–6.

112. Hermanides HK, Laheÿ-de Boer AM, Zuidmeer L, et al. Brassica oleracea pollen, a new source of occupational allergens. Allergy 2006;61(4):498–502.

113. Lee JY, Lee YD, Bahn JW, et al. A case of occupational asthma and rhinitis caused by Sanyak and Korean ginseng dusts. Allergy 2006;61(3):392–3.

114. Compes E, Bartolomé B, Fernández-Nieto M, et al. Occupational asthma from dried flowers of Carthamus tinctorious (safflower) and Achillea millefolium (yarrow). Allergy 2006;61(10):1239–40.

115. Vereda A, Quirce S, Fernández-Nieto M, et al. Occupational asthma due to spores of Pleurotus ostreatus. Allergy 2007;62(2):211–2.

116. Yates B, De Soyza A, Harkawat R, et al. Occupational asthma caused by Arabidopsis thaliana: a case of laboratory plant allergy. Eur Respir J 2008;32(4): 1111–2.

117. Vandenplas O, Pirson F, D'Alpaos V, et al. Occupational asthma caused by chamomile. Allergy 2008;63(8):1090–2.

118. Vandenplas O, D'Alpaos V, César M, et al. Occupational asthma caused by linseed oilcake. Allergy 2008;63(9):1250–1.

119. Vandenplas O, Sohy C, D'Alpaos V, et al. Tomato-induced occupational asthma in a greenhouse worker. J Allergy Clin Immunol 2008;122(6):1229–31.

Pathogenesis and Disease Mechanisms of Occupational Asthma

Zana L. Lummus, PhD[a], Adam V. Wisnewski, PhD[b],
David I. Bernstein, MD[c],*

KEYWORDS

- Occupational asthma • Airway hyperresponsiveness
- Workplace allergens • Immune mechanisms
- Airway remodeling • Oxidative stress • Genetic susceptibility

CLASSIFICATION OF OCCUPATIONAL ASTHMA

A generally accepted definition proposed in an authoritative text, *Asthma in the Workplace*,[1] has defined occupational asthma (OA) as "variable airflow limitation and/or airway hyperresponsiveness due to exposure to a specific causal agent present in a particular work environment and not to stimuli encountered outside the workplace." This definition of OA does not include workplace activation or exacerbation of preexisting asthma symptoms, which is called work-aggravated asthma. OA can be further subclassified into 2 different types:

- OA appearing after an asymptomatic latent period (during which immune sensitization is thought to develop), including (1) IgE-associated OA typically triggered by high–molecular weight (HMW) protein antigens and (2) IgE-independent OA typically triggered by low–molecular weight (LMW) chemicals (isocyanates, red cedar dust). This type is sometimes called immunologic OA.

This work was supported by Grant No. R01 OH008795 from the National Institute for Occupational Safety and Health/Centers for Disease Control.
The authors have nothing to disclose.
[a] Department of Internal Medicine, University of Cincinnati College of Medicine, 3255 Eden Avenue, Cincinnati, OH 45267-0563, USA
[b] Department of Internal Medicine, Yale School of Medicine, 333 Cedar Street, New Haven, CT 06510, USA
[c] Division of Immunology, Allergy and Rheumatology, University of Cincinnati College of Medicine, 3255 Eden Avenue, Cincinnati, OH 45267-0563, USA
* Corresponding author.
E-mail address: bernstdd@ucmail.uc.edu

- OA that appears after single or multiple workplace exposures to nonspecific irritants at a high concentration. The term reactive airways dysfunction syndrome (RADS) has been coined to describe this type of OA. This type is sometimes called nonimmunologic OA. RADS is covered in detail in another article by Brooks and Bernstein elsewhere in this issue.

CLINICAL MANIFESTATIONS OF OA
Symptoms and Degree of Severity

The clinical manifestations of OA are similar to those found in nonoccupational asthma, and patients present with varying degrees of disease severity. Patients with mild condition may experience only episodic dry cough, chest tightness, and increased breathing effort at work. In more severe cases, symptoms can include wheezing, cough, chest tightness, shortness of breath, and dyspnea that persist away from the work environment. Some individuals may develop bronchitis, nocturnal awakening, or concomitant symptoms of rhinoconjunctivitis.[2]

Airway Hyperresponsiveness

Nearly all individuals with asthma with active symptoms exhibit airway hyperresponsiveness (AHR), an exaggerated response to bronchoconstrictor stimuli, which can be assessed by pharmacologic testing (eg, methacholine inhalation challenge) or nonpharmacologic means (eg, exercise challenge). In the general population, only about 50% of individuals with AHR have symptoms of respiratory disease,[3] but it does appear to be a risk factor for asthma because it may precede development of asthma.[4,5] Although preexisting AHR does not consistently predict development of OA caused by a sensitizer, a link between AHR and active symptoms of OA is firmly established. Workers with OA often exhibit decreases or resolution of AHR corresponding with reduced or disappearance of symptoms after cessation of exposure to causative agents in the workplace.[6]

Patterns of Asthmatic Responses

Three patterns of asthmatic response in workers with OA have been defined from decreases in forced expiratory volume in the first second of expiration with time after antigen challenge during specific inhalation challenge (SIC) testing.[7] The isolated immediate or early-onset asthmatic reaction, which begins immediately and lasts for 1 to 2 hours, is characterized by smooth muscle contraction and/or edema and is not usually associated with inflammatory cells or increased AHR. Dual-phase asthmatic responses are characterized by both an early- and late-phase bronchoconstriction interrupted by a recovery interval with the late response occurring 3 to 12 hours after challenge. The isolated late-phase asthmatic response is almost always elicited by chemical sensitizers and, rarely, if ever associated with measurable specific IgE.[8] All late-phase responses to specific sensitizers are associated with infiltration of eosinophils, basophils, and/or neutrophils and increased AHR.

Chronic irreversible airflow obstruction observed in some workers with OA is believed to be associated with airway remodeling. Changes reflecting airway remodeling include loss of ciliated epithelial cells, increased mucous secretion by goblet cells, basement membrane thickening due to subepithelial fibrosis with fibroblast and myelofibroblast activation, and hypertrophy of airway smooth muscle cells.[6]

WORKPLACE SUBSTANCES PROVED TO BE CAUSATIVE AGENTS OF OA

Compendia of more than 250 specific causative agents can be found in other publications or on special Web sites,[9–12] and these agents can be generally subdivided based on size as HMW (>10,000 Da) or LMW (<1000 Da). HMW allergens are macromolecules capable of inducing a specific IgE antibody response and are usually associated with workplace sensitization to animals, plants, and/or microorganisms. For some of the HMW agents, major and minor allergens have been purified, characterized, and recombinantly cloned/expressed (eg, wheat proteins, cow dander). Of some 189 reported HMW allergens, 56% have been confirmed by bronchial provocation tests.

HMW allergens that cause OA may possess functional characteristics (eg, proteolytic activity) that promote their allergenicity.[13,14] Other HMW allergens (eg, house dust mites) possess pattern recognition receptors capable of stimulating innate immune responses via toll receptors, which may enhance their sensitizing potential.[15] Although most HMW occupational allergens are proteins, complex polysaccharides, such as those contained in vegetable gums, may also cause OA.

Approximately 78 LMW chemicals have been described as causes of OA. Prominent LMW sensitizers include diisocyanates, acid anhydrides, amines, metals, therapeutic drugs, and reactive dyes.[12] Structural modeling of these chemicals suggests that certain characteristics, particularly the presence of functional groups containing 2 or more reactive nitrogen or oxygen and the ability to conjugate with lysine, may be critical to OA pathogenesis.[16] The reactive functional groups of isocyanate and other LMW asthma-causing chemicals are known to covalently bind to self-macromolecules, especially airway proteins such as human serum albumin, causing conformational changes, including formation of new antigenic determinants capable of triggering immune sensitization.[17]

IMMUNE MECHANISMS THAT DRIVE THE INFLAMMATORY PROCESSES OF OA
IgE-Mediated Mechanisms

Specific IgE-mediated sensitization to a workplace antigen accounts for 90% of cases of OA.[18] In type I IgE-mediated hypersensitivity reactions, IgE antibodies bind to and cross-link mast cell receptors, leading to degranulation and release of mediators that elicit asthmatic reactions in susceptible individuals. Respiratory sensitization occurs by inhalation of the substance, uptake by antigen-presenting cells such as dendritic cells that process antigens, and migration of these cells to regional lymph nodes where antigen is presented to $CD4^+$ T helper (T_H) cells that initiate an immune response. The nature of the immune response is influenced by the cytokine milieu at the site of lymphocyte stimulation. Depending on host factors and the antigenic epitopes, T_H cells differentiate into subpopulations of effector cells that produce different cytokines. The 2 most polarized subsets are T_H1 and T_H2 cells. Interferon-γ is the principle effector cytokine produced by T_H1 cells, which promotes isotype switching of B cells to immunoglobulin isotypes associated with phagocyte-dependent host reactions. T_H2 cells produce 3 cytokines, interleukin (IL) 4, IL-5, and IL-13, shown to critically influence asthma pathogenesis in mouse models,[19] and the levels of all these are increased in asthmatic patients.[20] IL-4 is essential for differentiation and expansion of T_H2 cells by upregulating the transcription factor GATA-3 in naive T cells.[21] IL-4 (together with IL-13) also promotes isotype switching from IgM to IgE production[22] and promotes expression of both high- and low-affinity Fcε receptors.[23] IL-5 regulates airway eosinophilia in asthma by promoting eosinophil differentiation, recruitment, activation, and survival.[24] In addition to promoting isotype switching to IgE, IL-13 also acts on airway epithelial cells and smooth muscle cells to affect airway remodeling and development of AHR.[25] Despite the evidence linking these 3 cytokines to the pathogenesis of allergic bronchial asthma, clinical trials using neutralization of these cytokines for asthma immunotherapy have provided disappointing results.[26-28] It seems probable that human asthma involves a greater variety of phenotypic subtypes than those discovered in mouse models. There is substantial evidence implicating contributions of several other T_H subsets, including T_H9, T_H17, T_H25, as well as T_H1, T_H3, regulatory T cells, and invariant natural killer T cells to inflammatory processes contributing to asthma aggravation and pathogenesis.[29]

The main feature of chronic OA caused by the prototypic LMW chemical sensitizer, toluene diisocyanate (TDI), is airway inflammation.[30] Bronchial biopsy studies in workers with TDI asthma reveal a mixed infiltrate of activated T cells, eosinophils, neutrophils, and macrophages. Despite specific IgE being detectable in only a minority of cases of diisocyanate-induced asthma (DA), the histopathologic findings are indistinguishable from those observed in individuals with allergic asthma.[31–33] Bronchial biopsy results of workers after inhalation challenge with diisocyanates, however, failed to demonstrate expression of messenger RNA for IgE ε chains and IL-4, which is further evidence against a role for IgE in this type of OA.[34]

Cell-Mediated Immune Mechanisms

Alternative mechanisms have been invoked to explain chemically induced OA. Cell-mediated immunity or delayed-type hypersensitivity has been postulated as a possible mechanism for isocyanate asthma; however, scientific evidence for this hypothesis is lacking. Anecdotal cases of concomitant contact dermatitis and OA as a result of chemical causes of OA (eg, ammonium persulfate in hair dressers) have been reported.[35] In addition, delayed patch testing responses were not identified in a study of workers with DA.[36] In one small study, hexamethylene diisocyanate (HDI)-conjugated epithelial cell proteins stimulated proliferation of peripheral mononuclear cells from workers with DA but not HDI-exposed nonasthmatic subjects.[37] However, in vitro lymphocyte proliferative responses to diisocyanate antigens have not been rigorously validated as predictors of DA.

Innate Responses

Nonadaptive immune responses could play a role in chemically induced OA. Isocyanates may have intrinsic effects resulting in production of proinflammatory cytokines. For example, peripheral mononuclear cells challenged in vitro with diisocyanate-albumin conjugate antigens show enhanced release of histamine-releasing factors and β-chemokines, particularly monocyte chemoattractant protein 1 (MCP-1).[38] Furthermore, in vitro enhancement of diisocyanate-albumin conjugate–driven MCP-1 production by blood cells was found to be strongly associated with DA and served as a diagnostic marker, identifying 79% of workers with DA, with 91% specificity.[33] Wisnewski and colleagues[39] demonstrated that human peripheral blood mononuclear cells stimulated in vitro with HDI-albumin or control albumin antigens showed marked changes in gene/protein expression that seemed to be specific for the isocyanate moiety. Significant changes were noted in lysosomal genes, as well as increased expression of chemokines, including migration inhibitory factor and MCP-1, which attract mononuclear cells, chitinases (pattern recognition receptors), and oxidized low-density lipoprotein (CD68). Other investigators studied the gene expression profile of macrophages derived from the THP-1 human cell line and cultured with solubilized HDI and identified altered expression of genes involved in detoxification, oxidative stress, cytokine signaling, and apoptosis.[40] Thus, there is ample evidence suggesting that isocyanate chemicals stimulate nonadaptive immune responses that contribute to respiratory sensitization, airway inflammation, and clinical expression of OA.

Skin Exposure and OA

Although the respiratory tract has been the focus of most studies on OA, evidence is accumulating that the skin may also play an important role in pathogenesis as an exposure route for initiating immune sensitization.[41–50] This hypothesis of pathogenesis is similar to that of the atopic march and is supported by the identification of structural genes as determinants of severe atopic dermatitis, a condition associated with heightened asthma prevalence.[51–54] It is theorized that once immune sensitization occurs via the skin, secondary respiratory tract exposure to exceedingly low levels (which do not trigger responses in nonsensitized workers) elicits airway inflammation and asthma.[48]

Despite being long overlooked as a potential exposure route contributing to OA, the skin exposure is well recognized as a mechanism for inducing immune sensitization, including production of allergen-specific IgE molecules.[55,56] Uptake of small reactive chemicals as well as large protein molecules is well documented and thought to involve specific dendritic cell populations that reside in the epidermal as well as the dermal layers of skin.[57–59] Once skin dendritic cells become activated by allergen (to express appropriate receptors), a chemokine gradient directs them to draining lymph nodes.[60,61] The outcome of skin exposure varies for different chemicals. For example, skin exposure to some occupational chemicals induces strong T_H2-skewed responses, whereas others induce T_H1 skewed responses.[62–64] Exposure dose further influences the outcome of skin exposure, which may be nonlinear and/or paradoxically limited at higher doses.[45,47]

Increasing recognition of the potential for occupational skin exposure to contribute to OA has spawned the development of animal models to further investigate potential pathogenic mechanisms. Several different reports have confirmed the ability of major occupational allergens to induce systemic immune sensitization and exacerbate subsequent inflammatory responses to respiratory tract inflammation in animal models.[41,45–47,50] In many of these studies, skin exposure has been found to be more potent than respiratory tract exposure for eliciting primary immune sensitization, providing further support for an important role in disease prevention.

NONIMMUNOLOGIC MECHANISMS

Although the immune system clearly plays an important role in OA, it has been suggested that this response is a secondary phenomenon, rather than the underlying cause of disease.[65,66] It is theorized that the primary defect in asthma may relate to impaired barrier function of the epithelium, which allows greater access of environmental allergens, microorganisms, and toxicants, which in turn trigger allergic-type inflammation.[67–70] Impaired barrier function may be because of internal (genetic) or external (occupational exposure) factors that modulate the normal epithelial damage-repair cycle of the human airways.[71] A similar process has been shown to account for certain types of allergic skin disease (described earlier), supporting the overall concept of barrier defect–driven inflammation at epithelial cell surfaces.[72]

Epithelial Injury-Repair Cycle

The airway epithelium constitutes the interface between the internal milieu of the lung and the external environment. As the first point of contact for respirable particles, vapors, and aerosols, the airway epithelium is most susceptible to their damaging effects. As mentioned earlier, some compounds that cause OA are enzymes (eg, detergents/baking allergens) capable of directly disrupting cell-cell or cell-matrix interactions, whereas other occupational allergens are intrinsically cytotoxic (diisocyanates, anhydrides).[13,16,73–75] Damage to the airway epithelium stimulates cell turnover through a process that involves several autocrine growth factors as well as signals from the adjacent mesenchyme.[76,77] Epidermal growth factor, fibroblast growth factor, transforming growth factor β, and their corresponding receptors, have emerged as critical mediators in this process.[78–80] Increased expression of these and other growth factors (insulinlike growth factor, platelet-derived growth factor, nerve growth factor, vascular endothelial growth factor) is observed in the airway epithelium of patients with active asthma.[68,81,82] Continuing cycles of epithelial damage and repair, as might be caused by occupational exposures, may create a chronic wound scenario, which may increase the potential for the development of allergic sensitization.[68,83,84]

The Epithelial-Mesenchymal Trophic Unit

Opposing layers of epithelial and mesenchymal cells constitute trophic units in which the resident cells counterregulate each other's differentiation via secreted factors.[85–87] The area between these 2 cell layers contains extracellular matrix and a network of nerve fibers.[85] Dysregulation of the epithelial-mesenchymal trophic unit, in response to specific inhaled exposures, has been documented in nonhuman primate studies and postulated to explain pathologic changes associated with asthma, which occur at very early stages of disease.[88–90] The effects of specific occupational exposures on epithelial-mesenchymal interactions in vivo remain unstudied; however, in vitro studies suggest a possible influence on critical epithelial signaling components.[91,92]

Remodeling of the Airway Wall

It has been postulated that when epithelial injury and repair becomes a chronic cycle, the structure of the airway wall may become remodeled, further increasing the opportunity for tissue penetration by allergens/toxins/viruses.[93,94] Structural changes observed in OA include hyalinization/thickening of the laminar reticularis, increased numbers of myofibroblasts, and hypertrophy/metaplasia of smooth muscle and mucous cells, which may persist despite cessation of exposure.[95–98] In animal models, profibrotic cytokines, especially IL-13, mediate many of these changes.[99,100] The appearance of remodeling during the natural history of OA remains unclear. However, in patients with environmental asthma, such architectural changes occur early in the course of disease and may precede inflammatory changes.[101,102]

Toxicity

Many of the compounds that cause OA are cytotoxic at relatively low doses, including the LMW chemicals, isocyanates, acid anhydrides, acrylates, and certain metals.[74,103–105] The immune response to these compounds has generally been studied independent of their toxicity; however, an interrelationship between these effects may exist. The danger signals elicited by certain occupational exposures (or coexposures) may play an important role in the development of specific immune responses.[106–109]

Oxidative Stress

Several different studies provide evidence of increased oxidative stress during asthma, both locally within the airways as well as systemically.[110–112] Exhaled breath condensate and bronchoalveolar lavage samples from affected individuals have been shown to contain increased levels of 8-isoprostane and other well-established markers of oxidative stress.[113,114] Peripherally, additional biomarkers of oxidative stress (superoxide anion generation, lipid peroxidation, total nitrates/nitrites, total protein carbonyls, and total protein sulfhydryls) may be increased, concomitant with decreased levels of specific antioxidants (superoxide dismutase, catalase activity, glutathione, and glutathione peroxidase activity).[112,115,116] It remains unclear if increased levels of oxidative stress observed in asthmatic individuals is a cause of disease or rather a result of ongoing inflammation in the airways, which itself produces reactive oxygen species. Regardless of the source, oxidative stress is thought to aggravate asthmatic airway inflammation via multiple mechanisms, including proinflammatory mediators, and effects on smooth muscle and mucous secretion.[117–119]

The molecular mechanisms by which oxidative stress affects cellular responses are beginning to be deciphered. At low levels of oxidative stress, the transcription factor Nrf2 is released to the nucleus where it induces expression of more than 200 genes with antioxidant response elements in their promoters.[120] When oxidative stress exceeds the protective capacity of Nrf2-induced genes, additional intracellular cascades (MAPK pathway, nuclear factor $\kappa\beta$) may be triggered, leading eventually to the expression of proinflammatory cytokines, chemokines, and adhesion molecules.[117,121]

Certain exposures (diesel exhaust, ozone) are well recognized for their ability to induce oxidative stress and have been shown to act as adjuvants for the development of allergic-type respiratory responses in animal models.[122–126] Recent studies suggest that other important occupational exposures (isocyanates, chlorobenzene, cerium, and silicon oxide constituents of nanoparticles) may also induce oxidative stress.[74,127–131]

Thiol Redox Homeostasis

Thiols, especially glutathione, play a major role in protecting the airway against oxidant damage.[132,133] Airway fluid thiol levels are normally maintained at high levels (>100 μm), more than 10-fold more than systemic blood levels and are intimately connected to redox-sensitive (proinflammatory) intracellular signaling cascades.[134] In vivo animal models and in vitro studies with human cells have demonstrated that isocyanate chemicals have marked effects on airway thiols.[135,136] Glutathione may be an especially critical target because its levels are known to modulate T_H1 versus T_H2 priming by dendritic cells and subsequent asthmatic response in animal models.[137,138] Human genetic studies that associate glutathione-dependent enzyme polymorphisms (GST-P1, GST-M) with occupational and environmental asthma further support a potentially important role for airway thiols in asthma pathogenesis.[139,140]

Neurogenic Inflammation

The airway wall is entwined with fibers from neurons, some of which penetrate the basement membrane, reaching into the epithelial cell layer, where they sense external signals via specific receptors, and secrete factors capable of eliciting inflammation and bronchoconstriction.[141] Critical mediators include neuropeptides, substance P (SP), neurokinins (NKs), calcitonin gene-related peptides (GCRPs), and vasoactive intestinal peptides, which trigger responses from immune, vascular, and smooth muscle cells via specific receptors.[142–144] Further cross talk between neuronal and immune cells may be modulated through the epithelial-derived enzyme neutral endopeptidase (NEP), which breaks down proinflammatory neuropeptides.[145] Epithelial NEP activity can be further affected by occupational and/or environmental exposures.[146,147] Thus, neuronal cells produce potent mediators that may interact with other cell types to influence exposure-induced asthmatic responses.

A single neuronal receptor, TRPA1, which recognizes a wide variety of noxious stimuli, including occupational allergens (diisocyanates), environmental irritants (cigarette smoke, chlorine), and endogenous compounds (reactive oxygen/nitrogen species, arachidonic acid derivatives), has now been molecularly cloned.[148,149] In animal studies, TRPA1 expression colocalizes with SP, NK, and GCRP in nerve fibers in the airways, and TRPA1 knockout mice exhibit reduced inflammation in an ovalbumin asthma model.[150,151] However, species differences in TRPA1 activation, as well as general innervation of the lung, are well noted, limiting translation of animal studies on airway neuroinflammation to human asthma.[141,152]

GENETIC SUSCEPTIBILITY FACTORS FOR OA

OA syndromes, such as nonoccupational asthma, are likely polygenic disorders. Identification of specific genes that contribute to OA has been challenging because study populations are relatively smaller than those needed for genetic association studies. Genetic studies in OA to date can be categorized as those associated with immunoregulation and innate immunity and those associated with T_H2 immunity and antioxidant enzyme genes.

Genes Associated with Immunoregulation and Innate Immunity

Candidate gene studies have been reported investigating associations between HLA class II antigen alleles or haplotypes and isocyanate-induced OA. Bignon and colleagues[153] evaluated HLA class II DQA1, DQB1, DPB1, and DRB alleles and reported that confirmed DA was associated with DQB1*0503 and the allelic combination DQB1*0201/0301. The DQB1*0501 allele and the DQA1*0101-DQB1*0501-DR1 haplotype seemed to be protective because their levels were increased among healthy exposed controls and decreased in DA. These findings were confirmed in a second study.[154] Single amino acid substitutions at residue 57 of aspartic acid in DQB1*0503 was significantly increased in workers with DA and negatively associated with a valine substitution at DQB1*0501.[155] However, these findings were not reproducible in a smaller US study, a European study of DA, or a similar Korean study.[156,157] In the Korean study, HLA DRB1*1501-DQB1*0602-DPB1*0501 haplotype level was significantly increased in 84 workers with TDI asthma compared with 2 asymptomatic comparator groups.[157]

HLA associations have been identified with other chemical causes of OA. A higher frequency of HLA DQB1*0603 and DQB1*0302 alleles and a reduced frequency of the DQB1*0501 allele has been reported in western red cedar sawmill workers with DA when compared with healthy workers.[158] Among chemical workers exposed to acid anhydride chemical sensitizers, HLA class II allele DQB1(*)0501 within DQ5 HLA was associated with specific IgE to at least one acid anhydride antigen.[159]

A total of 335 research workers were genotyped for TLR4/8551 and TLR4/8851 single nucleotide polymorphism (SNP) variants, and it was found that workers with the TLR4 8851 G variant have reduced responsiveness to inhalation of endotoxin and were at higher risk for atopy and sensitization to laboratory animal allergens.[160]

T_H2 Gene Markers

T_H2 cytokine gene polymorphisms of IL-4 receptor alpha (IL4RA) and IL-13 have been associated with allergic asthma and/or allergic sensitization.[161] A candidate gene study was performed in 103 isocyanate-exposed workers with DA confirmed by a positive SIC test, 115 symptomatic workers with negative SIC tests, and 150 asymptomatic spray painters exposed to HDI. DNA was extracted, and workers were genotyped for IL4RA (I50V), IL4RA (Q551R), IL4RA (E375A), IL13 (R110Q), and CD14 (C159T) SNPs. The interactions between diisocyanate exposure (HDI vs methylene diphenyl diisocyanate, TDI) and specific genotype combinations (ie, IL4RA II + IL13 RR, IL4RA II + CD14 CT, and IL4RA II + IL13 RR + CD14 CT) were significantly associated with DA compared with SIC-negative workers. When comparing HDI-exposed workers with DA (n = 50) and a different comparison group of asymptomatic HDI-exposed workers (n = 150), the association between DA and the IL4RA II + CD14 CT and IL4RA II + IL13 RR + CD14 CT genotype combinations trended toward statistical significance ($P<.10$) after adjustment for relevant confounding variables.[161–163]

Antioxidant Enzyme Genes

Gene SNPs associated with the mu, theta, and pi classes of the glutathione-S-transferase (GST) isoenzyme superfamily have been studied as predictors of DA. There is good rationale to explore GST genotype variants in that GST has been shown to modify biotransformation of isocyanates and excretion of metabolic products.[164] Reduced glutathione directly inhibits in vitro binding of diisocyanates with albumin.[165] Deletion of the GSTM1 gene (null genotype) has been associated with a 2-fold increased risk of DA.[140] The GSTP1 Val/Val homozygous genotype was lower in DA, suggesting a protective modifying effect (odds ratio, 0.23; $P = .074$).[139]

Genome-wide association studies have not been performed extensively in OA. Recently, groups of Korean workers including 84 with TDI asthma and 263 unexposed controls underwent genotyping with GeneChip arrays consisting of 500,000 SNPs.[166] Several SNPs of the α-T-catenin (CTNNA3) gene were identified to be significantly associated with DA. CTNNA3 is a molecule involved in E-cadherin–mediated cellular adhesion. The significance of this finding is unknown.

SUMMARY

OA is one of the most common forms of work-related lung disease in all industrialized nations. The clinical management of patients with OA depends on an understanding of the multifactorial pathogenetic mechanisms that can contribute to this disease. Once established, the clinical manifestations of OA are similar to those found in nonoccupational adult asthma, but the unique relationship of OA to a specific workplace antigen offers the possibility of successful therapy by early diagnosis and cessation of exposure to the causative agent. Specific IgE-mediated sensitization to HMW antigens accounts for 90% of cases of OA. LMW chemical sensitizers have generally not been found to cause OA by an IgE-mediated mechanism. Numerous factors have been found to contribute to the pathogenesis of chemically induced OA, including innate immune mechanisms and nonimmunologic mechanisms of epithelial injury, airway remodeling, oxidative stress, neurogenic inflammation, and genetic risk factors. Genes found to be associated with increased susceptibility to OA include HLA class II genes, genes associated with innate immunity and T_H2 immunity, and antioxidant enzyme genes.

REFERENCES

1. Bernstein IL, Bernstein DI, Chan-Yeung M, et al. Definition and classification of asthma. In: Bernstein IL, Chan-Yeung M, Malo JL, et al, editors. Asthma in the workplace. 3rd edition. New York: Taylor & Francis Group; 2006. p. 1–8.
2. Lombardo LJ, Balmes JR. Occupational asthma: a review. Environ Health Perspect 2000;108(Suppl 4):697–704.
3. Cockroft DW, Bercheid BA, Murdock KY. Unimodal distribution of bronchial hyperresponsiveness to inhaled histamine in a random population. Chest 1983;8:751–4.
4. Hopp RJ, Townley RG, Biven RE, et al. The presence of airway reactivity before the development of asthma. Am Rev Respir Dis 1990;141:2–8.

5. Laprise C, Laviolette M, Boutet M, et al. Asymptomatic airway hyperresponsiveness: relationships with airway inflammation and remodelling. Eur Respir J 1999; 14:63–73.
6. Maestrelli P, Fabbri LM, Mapp CE. Pathophysiology. In: Bernstein IL, Chan-Yeung M, Malo JL, et al, editors. Asthma in the workplace. 3rd edition. New York: Taylor & Francis Group; 2006. p. 109–40.
7. Vandenplas O, Malo JL. Inhalation challenges with agents causing occupational asthma. Eur Respir J 1997;10:2612–29.
8. Perrin B, Cartier A, Ghezzo H, et al. Reassessment of the temporal patterns of bronchial obstruction after exposure to occupational sensitizing agents. J Allergy Clin Immunol 1991;87:630–9.
9. Bardana EJ Jr. 10. Occupational asthma. J Allergy Clin Immunol 2008;121: S408–11.
10. Dykewicz MS. Occupational asthma: current concepts in pathogenesis, diagnosis, and management. J Allergy Clin Immunol 2009;123:519–28.
11. Quirce S, Sastre J. New causes of occupational asthma. Curr Opin Allergy Clin Immunol 2011;11:80–5.
12. Malo J-L, Chan-Yeung M. Agents causing occupational asthma with key references. In: Bernstein IL, Chan-Yeung M, Malo JL, et al, editors. Asthma in the workplace. 3rd edition. New York: Taylor and Francis Group; 2006. p. 825–66.
13. Schweigert MK, Mackenzie DP, Sarlo K. Occupational asthma and allergy associated with the use of enzymes in the detergent industry—a review of the epidemiology, toxicology and methods of prevention. Clin Exp Allergy 2000;30: 1511–8.
14. Jacquet A. Interactions of airway epithelium with protease allergens in the allergic response. Clin Exp Allergy 2011;41:305–11.
15. Nathan AT, Peterson EA, Chakir J, et al. Innate immune responses of airway epithelium to house dust mite are mediated through beta-glucan-dependent pathways. J Allergy Clin Immunol 2009;123:612–8.
16. Jarvis J, Seed MJ, Elton R, et al. Relationship between chemical structure and the occupational asthma hazard of low molecular weight organic compounds. Occup Environ Med 2005;62:243–50.
17. Zeiss CR, Levitz D, Chacon R, et al. Quantitation and new antigenic determinant specificity of antibodies induced by inhalation of trimellitic anhydride in man. Int Arch Allergy Appl Immunol 1980;61:380–8.
18. Tarlo SM, Liss GM. Occupational asthma: an approach to diagnosis and management. CMAJ 2003;168:867–71.
19. Wegmann M, Hauber HP. Experimental approaches towards allergic asthma therapy-murine asthma models. Recent Pat Inflamm Allergy Drug Discov 2010;4:37–53.
20. Wegmann M. Th2 cells as targets for therapeutic intervention in allergic bronchial asthma. Expert Rev Mol Diagn 2009;9:85–100.
21. Messi M, Giacchetto I, Nagata K, et al. Memory and flexibility of cytokine gene expression as separable properties of human T(H)1 and T(H)2 lymphocytes. Nat Immunol 2003;4:78–86.
22. Bacharier LB, Geha RS. Molecular mechanisms of IgE regulation. J Allergy Clin Immunol 2000;105:S547–58.
23. Renauld JC. New insights into the role of cytokines in asthma. J Clin Pathol 2001;54:577–89.
24. Rosenberg HF, Phipps S, Foster PS. Eosinophil trafficking in allergy and asthma. J Allergy Clin Immunol 2007;119:1303–10 [quiz: 1311–2].

25. Wills-Karp M. Interleukin-13 in asthma pathogenesis. Immunol Rev 2004;202: 175–90.
26. Borish LC, Nelson HS, Lanz MJ, et al. Interleukin-4 receptor in moderate atopic asthma. A phase I/II randomized, placebo-controlled trial. Am J Respir Crit Care Med 1999;160:1816–23.
27. Leckie MJ, ten Brinke A, Khan J, et al. Effects of an interleukin-5 blocking monoclonal antibody on eosinophils, airway hyper-responsiveness, and the late asthmatic response. Lancet 2000;356:2144–8.
28. Wenzel S, Wilbraham D, Fuller R, et al. Effect of an interleukin-4 variant on late phase asthmatic response to allergen challenge in asthmatic patients: results of two phase 2a studies. Lancet 2007;370:1422–31.
29. Vock C, Hauber HP, Wegmann M. The other T helper cells in asthma pathogenesis. J Allergy (Cairo) 2010;2010: Article ID 519298, 14.
30. Hargreave FE, Ramsdale EH, Kirby JG, et al. Asthma and the role of inflammation. Eur J Respir Dis Suppl 1986;147:16–21.
31. Cartier A, Grammer L, Malo JL, et al. Specific serum antibodies against isocyanates: association with occupational asthma. J Allergy Clin Immunol 1989;84:507–14.
32. Bentley AM, Maestrelli P, Saetta M, et al. Activated T-lymphocytes and eosinophils in the bronchial mucosa in isocyanate-induced asthma. J Allergy Clin Immunol 1992;89:821–9.
33. Bernstein DI, Cartier A, Cote J, et al. Diisocyanate antigen-stimulated monocyte chemoattractant protein-1 synthesis has greater test efficiency than specific antibodies for identification of diisocyanate asthma. Am J Respir Crit Care Med 2002;166:445–50.
34. Jones MG, Floyd A, Nouri-Aria KT, et al. Is occupational asthma to diisocyanates a non-IgE-mediated disease? J Allergy Clin Immunol 2006;117:663–9.
35. Yawalkar N, Helbling A, Pichler CE, et al. T cell involvement in persulfate triggered occupational contact dermatitis and asthma. Ann Allergy Asthma Immunol 1999;82:401–4.
36. Kanerva L, Estlander T, Jolanki R, et al. Asthma from diisocyanates is not mediated through a Type IV, patch-test-positive mechanism. Contact Dermatitis 2001;44:247.
37. Wisnewski AV, Lemus R, Karol MH, et al. Isocyanate-conjugated human lung epithelial cell proteins: a link between exposure and asthma? J Allergy Clin Immunol 1999;104:341–7.
38. Lummus ZL, Alam R, Bernstein JA, et al. Diisocyanate antigen-enhanced production of monocyte chemoattractant protein-1, IL-8, and tumor necrosis factor-alpha by peripheral mononuclear cells of workers with occupational asthma. J Allergy Clin Immunol 1998;102:265–74.
39. Wisnewski AV, Liu Q, Liu J, et al. Human innate immune responses to hexamethylene diisocyanate (HDI) and HDI-albumin conjugates. Clin Exp Allergy 2008;38:957–67.
40. Verstraelen S, Wens B, Hooyberghs J, et al. Gene expression profiling of in vitro cultured macrophages after exposure to the respiratory sensitizer hexamethylene diisocyanate. Toxicol In Vitro 2008;22:1107–14.
41. Ban M, Morel G, Langonne I, et al. TDI can induce respiratory allergy with Th2-dominated response in mice. Toxicology 2006;218:39–47.
42. Jang AS, Choi IS, Koh YI, et al. Increase in airway hyperresponsiveness among workers exposed to methylene diphenyldiisocyanate compared to workers exposed to toluene diisocyanate at a petrochemical plant in Korea. Am J Ind Med 2000;37:663–7.

43. Pauluhn J, Poole A. Brown Norway rat asthma model of diphenylmethane-4,4'-diisocyanate (MDI): determination of the elicitation threshold concentration of after inhalation sensitization. Toxicology 2011;281:15–24.

44. Scheerens H, Buckley TL, Muis TL, et al. Long-term topical exposure to toluene diisocyanate in mice leads to antibody production and in vivo airway hyperresponsiveness three hours after intranasal challenge. Am J Respir Crit Care Med 1999;159:1074–80.

45. Wisnewski AV, Xu L, Robinson E, et al. Immune sensitization to methylene diphenyl diisocyanate (MDI) resulting from skin exposure: albumin as a carrier protein connecting skin exposure to subsequent respiratory responses. J Occup Med Toxicol 2011;6:6.

46. Vanoirbeek JA, Tarkowski M, Ceuppens JL, et al. Respiratory response to toluene diisocyanate depends on prior frequency and concentration of dermal sensitization in mice. Toxicol Sci 2004;80:310–21.

47. Herrick CA, Xu L, Wisnewski AV, et al. A novel mouse model of diisocyanate-induced asthma showing allergic-type inflammation in the lung after inhaled antigen challenge. J Allergy Clin Immunol 2002;109:873–8.

48. Bello D, Herrick CA, Smith TJ, et al. Skin exposure to isocyanates: reasons for concern. Environ Health Perspect 2007;115:328–35.

49. Redlich CA. Skin exposure and asthma: is there a connection? Proc Am Thorac Soc 2010;7:134–7.

50. Zhang XD, Fedan JS, Lewis DM, et al. Asthmalike biphasic airway responses in Brown Norway rats sensitized by dermal exposure to dry trimellitic anhydride powder. J Allergy Clin Immunol 2004;113:320–6.

51. Marenholz I, Nickel R, Ruschendorf F, et al. Filaggrin loss-of-function mutations predispose to phenotypes involved in the atopic march. J Allergy Clin Immunol 2006;118:866–71.

52. Spergel JM. From atopic dermatitis to asthma: the atopic march. Ann Allergy Asthma Immunol 2010;105:99–106 [quiz: 107–9, 117].

53. Spergel JM, Paller AS. Atopic dermatitis and the atopic march. J Allergy Clin Immunol 2003;112:S118–27.

54. Zheng T, Yu J, Oh MH, et al. The atopic march: progression from atopic dermatitis to allergic rhinitis and asthma. Allergy Asthma Immunol Res 2011;3:67–73.

55. Beck LA, Leung DY. Allergen sensitization through the skin induces systemic allergic responses. J Allergy Clin Immunol 2000;106:S258–63.

56. Herrick CA, MacLeod H, Glusac E, et al. Th2 responses induced by epicutaneous or inhalational protein exposure are differentially dependent on IL-4. J Clin Invest 2000;105:765–75.

57. Larregina AT, Falo LD Jr. Changing paradigms in cutaneous immunology: adapting with dendritic cells. J Invest Dermatol 2005;124:1–12.

58. Merad M, Ginhoux F, Collin M. Origin, homeostasis and function of Langerhans cells and other langerin-expressing dendritic cells. Nat Rev Immunol 2008;8:935–47.

59. Toebak MJ, Gibbs S, Bruynzeel DP, et al. Dendritic cells: biology of the skin. Contact Dermatitis 2009;60:2–20.

60. Martln-Fontecha A, Sebastiani S, Hopken UE, et al. Regulation of dendritic cell migration to the draining lymph node: impact on T lymphocyte traffic and priming. J Exp Med 2003;198:615–21.

61. Ohl L, Mohaupt M, Czeloth N, et al. CCR7 governs skin dendritic cell migration under inflammatory and steady-state conditions. Immunity 2004;21:279–88.

62. Dearman RJ, Moussavi A, Kemeny DM, et al. Contribution of CD4+ and CD8+ T lymphocyte subsets to the cytokine secretion patterns induced in mice during

sensitization to contact and respiratory chemical allergens. Immunology 1996; 89:502–10.

63. Hayashi M, Higashi K, Kato H, et al. Assessment of preferential Th1 or Th2 induction by low-molecular-weight compounds using a reverse transcription-polymerase chain reaction method: comparison of two mouse strains, C57BL/6 and BALB/c. Toxicol Appl Pharmacol 2001;177:38–45.

64. Vanoirbeek JA, Tarkowski M, Vanhooren HM, et al. Validation of a mouse model of chemical-induced asthma using trimellitic anhydride, a respiratory sensitizer, and dinitrochlorobenzene, a dermal sensitizer. J Allergy Clin Immunol 2006;117:1090–7.

65. Holgate ST. Has the time come to rethink the pathogenesis of asthma? Curr Opin Allergy Clin Immunol 2010;10:48–53.

66. Holgate ST. The airway epithelium is central to the pathogenesis of asthma. Allergol Int 2008;57:1–10.

67. Holgate ST, Roberts G, Arshad HS, et al. The role of the airway epithelium and its interaction with environmental factors in asthma pathogenesis. Proc Am Thorac Soc 2009;6:655–9.

68. Holgate ST. Epithelial damage and response. Clin Exp Allergy 2000;30(Suppl 1): 37–41.

69. Holgate ST, Lackie P, Wilson S, et al. Bronchial epithelium as a key regulator of airway allergen sensitization and remodeling in asthma. Am J Respir Crit Care Med 2000;162:S113–7.

70. Holgate ST, Lackie PM, Davies DE, et al. The bronchial epithelium as a key regulator of airway inflammation and remodelling in asthma. Clin Exp Allergy 1999; 29(Suppl 2):90–5.

71. Holgate ST, Davies DE, Powell RM, et al. Local genetic and environmental factors in asthma disease pathogenesis: chronicity and persistence mechanisms. Eur Respir J 2007;29:793–803.

72. Cookson W. The immunogenetics of asthma and eczema: a new focus on the epithelium. Nat Rev Immunol 2004;4:978–88.

73. Pons F, Fischer A, Frossard N, et al. Effect of toluene diisocyanate and its corresponding amines on viability and growth of human lung fibroblasts in culture. Cell Biol Toxicol 1999;15:333–40.

74. Wisnewski AV, Liu Q, Miller JJ, et al. Effects of hexamethylene diisocyanate exposure on human airway epithelial cells: in vitro cellular and molecular studies. Environ Health Perspect 2002;110:901–7.

75. Valdivieso R, Subiza J, Subiza JL, et al. Bakers' asthma caused by alpha amylase. Ann Allergy 1994;73:337–42.

76. Erjefalt JS, Persson CG. Airway epithelial repair: breathtakingly quick and multipotentially pathogenic. Thorax 1997;52:1010–2.

77. Zahm JM, Chevillard M, Puchelle E. Wound repair of human surface respiratory epithelium. Am J Respir Cell Mol Biol 1991;5:242–8.

78. Amishima M, Munakata M, Nasuhara Y, et al. Expression of epidermal growth factor and epidermal growth factor receptor immunoreactivity in the asthmatic human airway. Am J Respir Crit Care Med 1998;157:1907–12.

79. Davies DE, Polosa R, Puddicombe SM, et al. The epidermal growth factor receptor and its ligand family: their potential role in repair and remodelling in asthma. Allergy 1999;54:771–83.

80. Puddicombe SM, Polosa R, Richter A, et al. Involvement of the epidermal growth factor receptor in epithelial repair in asthma. FASEB J 2000;14:1362–74.

81. Hoshino M, Takahashi M, Aoike N. Expression of vascular endothelial growth factor, basic fibroblast growth factor, and angiogenin immunoreactivity in

asthmatic airways and its relationship to angiogenesis. J Allergy Clin Immunol 2001;107:295–301.

82. Vignola AM, Chanez P, Chiappara G, et al. Transforming growth factor-beta expression in mucosal biopsies in asthma and chronic bronchitis. Am J Respir Crit Care Med 1997;156:591–9.

83. Hackett TL, Knight DA. The role of epithelial injury and repair in the origins of asthma. Curr Opin Allergy Clin Immunol 2007;7:63–8.

84. Davies DE, Holgate ST. Asthma: the importance of epithelial mesenchymal communication in pathogenesis. Inflammation and the airway epithelium in asthma. Int J Biochem Cell Biol 2002;34:1520–6.

85. Evans MJ, Van Winkle LS, Fanucchi MV, et al. The attenuated fibroblast sheath of the respiratory tract epithelial-mesenchymal trophic unit. Am J Respir Cell Mol Biol 1999;21:655–7.

86. Minoo P, King RJ. Epithelial-mesenchymal interactions in lung development. Annu Rev Physiol 1994;56:13–45.

87. Araya J, Cambier S, Morris A, et al. Integrin-mediated transforming growth factor-beta activation regulates homeostasis of the pulmonary epithelial-mesenchymal trophic unit. Am J Pathol 2006;169:405–15.

88. Joad JP, Kott KS, Bric JM, et al. Structural and functional localization of airway effects from episodic exposure of infant monkeys to allergen and/or ozone. Toxicol Appl Pharmacol 2006;214:237–43.

89. Plopper CG, Smiley-Jewell SM, Miller LA, et al. Asthma/allergic airways disease: does postnatal exposure to environmental toxicants promote airway pathobiology? Toxicol Pathol 2007;35:97–110.

90. Evans MJ, Fanucchi MV, Baker GL, et al. Atypical development of the tracheal basement membrane zone of infant rhesus monkeys exposed to ozone and allergen. Am J Physiol Lung Cell Mol Physiol 2003;285:L931–39.

91. Ogawa H, Inoue S, Ogushi F, et al. Toluene diisocyanate (TDI) induces production of inflammatory cytokines and chemokines by bronchial epithelial cells via the epidermal growth factor receptor and p38 mitogen-activated protein kinase pathways. Exp Lung Res 2006;32:245–62.

92. Zhang L, Rice AB, Adler K, et al. Vanadium stimulates human bronchial epithelial cells to produce heparin-binding epidermal growth factor-like growth factor: a mitogen for lung fibroblasts. Am J Respir Cell Mol Biol 2001;24:123–31.

93. Holgate ST. Epithelium dysfunction in asthma. J Allergy Clin Immunol 2007;120: 1233–44 [quiz: 1245–6].

94. Davies DE, Wicks J, Powell RM, et al. Airway remodeling in asthma: new insights. J Allergy Clin Immunol 2003;111:215–25 [quiz: 226].

95. Saetta M, Maestrelli P, Turato G, et al. Airway wall remodeling after cessation of exposure to isocyanates in sensitized asthmatic subjects. Am J Respir Crit Care Med 1995;151:489–94.

96. Mapp CE, Saetta M, Maestrelli P, et al. Mechanisms and pathology of occupational asthma. Eur Respir J 1994;7:544–54.

97. Paggiaro P, Bacci E, Paoletti P, et al. Bronchoalveolar lavage and morphology of the airways after cessation of exposure in asthmatic subjects sensitized to toluene diisocyanate. Chest 1990;98:536–42.

98. Saetta M, Di Stefano A, Maestrelli P, et al. Airway mucosal inflammation in occupational asthma induced by toluene diisocyanate. Am Rev Respir Dis 1992;145: 160–8.

99. Zhu Z, Zheng T, Homer RJ, et al. Acidic mammalian chitinase in asthmatic Th2 inflammation and IL-13 pathway activation. Science 2004;304:1678–82.

100. Elias JA, Zheng T, Lee CG, et al. Transgenic modeling of interleukin-13 in the lung. Chest 2003;123:339S–45S.
101. Barbato A, Turato G, Baraldo S, et al. Epithelial damage and angiogenesis in the airways of children with asthma. Am J Respir Crit Care Med 2006;174:975–81.
102. Fedorov IA, Wilson SJ, Davies DE, et al. Epithelial stress and structural remodelling in childhood asthma. Thorax 2005;60:389–94.
103. Venables KM. Low molecular weight chemicals, hypersensitivity, and direct toxicity: the acid anhydrides. Br J Ind Med 1989;46:222–32.
104. Autian J. Structure-toxicity relationships of acrylic monomers. Environ Health Perspect 1975;11:141–52.
105. Waters MD, Vaughan TO, Abernethy DJ, et al. Toxicity of platinum (IV) salts for cells of pulmonary origin. Environ Health Perspect 1975;12:45–56.
106. Willart MA, Lambrecht BN. The danger within: endogenous danger signals, atopy and asthma. Clin Exp Allergy 2009;39:12–9.
107. Gallucci S, Matzinger P. Danger signals: SOS to the immune system. Curr Opin Immunol 2001;13:114–9.
108. Lotze MT, Deisseroth A, Rubartelli A. Damage associated molecular pattern molecules. Clin Immunol 2007;124:1–4.
109. Seong SY, Matzinger P. Hydrophobicity: an ancient damage-associated molecular pattern that initiates innate immune responses. Nat Rev Immunol 2004;4:469–78.
110. Riedl MA, Nel AE. Importance of oxidative stress in the pathogenesis and treatment of asthma. Curr Opin Allergy Clin Immunol 2008;8:49–56.
111. Dozor AJ. The role of oxidative stress in the pathogenesis and treatment of asthma. Ann N Y Acad Sci 2010;1203:133–7.
112. Nadeem A, Raj HG, Chhabra SK. Increased oxidative stress in acute exacerbations of asthma. J Asthma 2005;42:45–50.
113. Loukides S, Bouros D, Papatheodorou G, et al. The relationships among hydrogen peroxide in expired breath condensate, airway inflammation, and asthma severity. Chest 2002;121:338–46.
114. Montuschi P, Corradi M, Ciabattoni G, et al. Increased 8-isoprostane, a marker of oxidative stress, in exhaled condensate of asthma patients. Am J Respir Crit Care Med 1999;160:216–20.
115. Suzuki S, Matsukura S, Takeuchi H, et al. Increase in reactive oxygen metabolite level in acute exacerbations of asthma. Int Arch Allergy Immunol 2008;146(Suppl 1):67–72.
116. Garcia-Larsen V, Chinn S, Rodrigo R, et al. Relationship between oxidative stress-related biomarkers and antioxidant status with asthma and atopy in young adults: a population-based study. Clin Exp Allergy 2009;39:379–86.
117. Janssen-Heininger YM, Poynter ME, Aesif SW, et al. Nuclear factor kappaB, airway epithelium, and asthma: avenues for redox control. Proc Am Thorac Soc 2009;6:249–55.
118. Fischer B, Voynow J. Neutrophil elastase induces MUC5AC messenger RNA expression by an oxidant-dependent mechanism. Chest 2000;117:317S–20S.
119. Kojima K, Kume H, Ito S, et al. Direct effects of hydrogen peroxide on airway smooth muscle tone: roles of $Ca2+$ influx and Rho-kinase. Eur J Pharmacol 2007;556:151–6.
120. Kaspar JW, Niture SK, Jaiswal AK. Nrf2:INrf2 (Keap1) signaling in oxidative stress. Free Radic Biol Med 2009;47:1304–9.
121. Rahman I. Oxidative stress and gene transcription in asthma and chronic obstructive pulmonary disease: antioxidant therapeutic targets. Curr Drug Targets Inflamm Allergy 2002;1:291–315.

122. Chan RC, Wang M, Li N, et al. Pro-oxidative diesel exhaust particle chemicals inhibit LPS-induced dendritic cell responses involved in T-helper differentiation. J Allergy Clin Immunol 2006;118:455–65.
123. Pacheco KA, Tarkowski M, Sterritt C, et al. The influence of diesel exhaust particles on mononuclear phagocytic cell-derived cytokines: IL-10, TGF-beta and IL-1 beta. Clin Exp Immunol 2001;126:374–83.
124. Corradi M, Alinovi R, Goldoni M, et al. Biomarkers of oxidative stress after controlled human exposure to ozone. Toxicol Lett 2002;134:219–25.
125. Wang J, Wang S, Manzer R, et al. Ozone induces oxidative stress in rat alveolar type II and type I-like cells. Free Radic Biol Med 2006;40:1914–28.
126. Backus-Hazzard GS, Howden R, Kleeberger SR. Genetic susceptibility to ozone-induced lung inflammation in animal models of asthma. Curr Opin Allergy Clin Immunol 2004;4:349–53.
127. Lee CT, Ylostalo J, Friedman M, et al. Gene expression profiling in mouse lung following polymeric hexamethylene diisocyanate exposure. Toxicol Appl Pharmacol 2005;205:53–64.
128. Kim SH, Choi GS, Ye YM, et al. Toluene diisocyanate (TDI) regulates haem oxygenase-1/ferritin expression: implications for toluene diisocyanate-induced asthma. Clin Exp Immunol 2010;160:489–97.
129. Eom HJ, Choi J. Oxidative stress of CeO2 nanoparticles via p38-Nrf-2 signaling pathway in human bronchial epithelial cell, Beas-2B. Toxicol Lett 2009;187:77–83.
130. Eom HJ, Choi J. Oxidative stress of silica nanoparticles in human bronchial epithelial cell, Beas-2B. Toxicol In Vitro 2009;23:1326–32.
131. Feltens R, Mogel I, Roder-Stolinski C, et al. Chlorobenzene induces oxidative stress in human lung epithelial cells in vitro. Toxicol Appl Pharmacol 2010; 242:100–8.
132. Reynaert NL. Glutathione biochemistry in asthma. Biochim Biophys Acta 2011. [Epub ahead of print].
133. Biswas SK, Rahman I. Environmental toxicity, redox signaling and lung inflammation: the role of glutathione. Mol Aspects Med 2009;30:60–76.
134. Fitzpatrick AM, Teague WG, Holguin F, et al. Airway glutathione homeostasis is altered in children with severe asthma: evidence for oxidant stress. J Allergy Clin Immunol 2009;123:146.e8–52.e8.
135. Lange RW, Day BW, Lemus R, et al. Intracellular S-glutathionyl adducts in murine lung and human bronchoepithelial cells after exposure to diisocyanato-toluene. Chem Res Toxicol 1999;12:931–6.
136. Lantz RC, Lemus R, Lange RW, et al. Rapid reduction of intracellular glutathione in human bronchial epithelial cells exposed to occupational levels of toluene diisocyanate. Toxicol Sci 2001;60:348–55.
137. Koike Y, Hisada T, Utsugi M, et al. Glutathione redox regulates airway hyperresponsiveness and airway inflammation in mice. Am J Respir Cell Mol Biol 2007; 37:322–9.
138. Peterson JD, Herzenberg LA, Vasquez K, et al. Glutathione levels in antigen-presenting cells modulate Th1 versus Th2 response patterns. Proc Natl Acad Sci U S A 1998;95:3071–6.
139. Mapp CE, Fryer AA, De Marzo N, et al. Glutathione S-transferase GSTP1 is a susceptibility gene for occupational asthma induced by isocyanates. J Allergy Clin Immunol 2002;109:867–72.
140. Piirila P, Wikman H, Luukkonen R, et al. Glutathione S-transferase genotypes and allergic responses to diisocyanate exposure. Pharmacogenetics 2001;11: 437–45.

141. van der Velden VH, Hulsmann AR. Autonomic innervation of human airways: structure, function, and pathophysiology in asthma. Neuroimmunomodulation 1999;6:145–59.

142. Barnes PJ. Neurogenic inflammation and asthma. J Asthma 1992;29:165–80.

143. Butler CA, Heaney LG. Neurogenic inflammation and asthma. Inflamm Allergy Drug Targets 2007;6:127–32.

144. Pisi G, Olivieri D, Chetta A. The airway neurogenic inflammation: clinical and pharmacological implications. Inflamm Allergy Drug Targets 2009;8:176–81.

145. Di Maria GU, Bellofiore S, Geppetti P. Regulation of airway neurogenic inflammation by neutral endopeptidase. Eur Respir J 1998;12:1454–62.

146. Gagnaire F, Ban M, Cour C, et al. Role of tachykinins and neutral endopeptidase in toluene diisocyanate-induced bronchial hyperresponsiveness in guinea pigs. Toxicology 1997;116:17–26.

147. Sheppard D, Thompson JE, Scypinski L, et al. Toluene diisocyanate increases airway responsiveness to substance P and decreases airway neutral endopeptidase. J Clin Invest 1988;81:1111–5.

148. Bessac BF, Jordt SE. Sensory detection and responses to toxic gases: mechanisms, health effects, and countermeasures. Proc Am Thorac Soc 2010;7: 269–77.

149. Bessac BF, Sivula M, von Hehn CA, et al. Transient receptor potential ankyrin 1 antagonists block the noxious effects of toxic industrial isocyanates and tear gases. FASEB J 2009;23:1102–14.

150. Nassenstein C, Kwong K, Taylor-Clark T, et al. Expression and function of the ion channel TRPA1 in vagal afferent nerves innervating mouse lungs. J Physiol 2008;586:1595–604.

151. Caceres AI, Brackmann M, Elia MD, et al. A sensory neuronal ion channel essential for airway inflammation and hyperreactivity in asthma. Proc Natl Acad Sci U S A 2009;106:9099–104.

152. Chen J, Kym PR. TRPA1: the species difference. J Gen Physiol 2009;133:623–5.

153. Bignon JS, Aron Y, Ju LY, et al. HLA class II alleles in isocyanate-induced asthma. Am J Respir Crit Care Med 1994;149:71–5.

154. Mapp CE, Beghe B, Balboni A, et al. Association between HLA genes and susceptibility to toluene diisocyanate-induced asthma. Clin Exp Allergy 2000; 30:651–6.

155. Balboni A, Baricordi OR, Fabbri LM, et al. Association between toluene diisocyanate-induced asthma and DQB1 markers: a possible role for aspartic acid at position 57. Eur Respir J 1996;9:207–10.

156. Beghe B, Padoan M, Moss CT, et al. Lack of association of HLA class I genes and TNF alpha-308 polymorphism in toluene diisocyanate-induced asthma. Allergy 2004;59:61–4.

157. Choi JH, Lee KW, Kim CW, et al. The HLA DRB1*1501-DQB1*0602-DPB1*0501 haplotype is a risk factor for toluene diisocyanate-induced occupational asthma. Int Arch Allergy Immunol 2009;150:156–63.

158. Horne C, Quintana PJ, Keown PA, et al. Distribution of DRB1 and DQB1 HLA class II alleles in occupational asthma due to western red cedar. Eur Respir J 2000;15:911–4.

159. Jones MG, Nielsen J, Welch J, et al. Association of HLA-DQ5 and HLA-DR1 with sensitization to organic acid anhydrides. Clin Exp Allergy 2004;34:812–6.

160. Pacheco K, Maier L, Silveira L, et al. Association of toll-like receptor 4 alleles with symptoms and sensitization to laboratory animals. J Allergy Clin Immunol 2008;122:896–902.e4.

161. Bernstein DI, Wang N, Campo P, et al. Diisocyanate asthma and gene-environment interactions with IL4RA, CD-14, and IL-13 genes. Ann Allergy Asthma Immunol 2006;97:800–6.

162. Bernstein DI, Kissling GE, Khurana Hershey G, et al. Hexamethylene diisocyanate asthma is associated with genetic polymorphisms of CD14, IL-13, and IL-4 receptor alpha. J Allergy Clin Immunol 2011;128:418–20.

163. Bernstein DI. Genetics of occupational asthma. Curr Opin Allergy Clin Immunol 2011;11:86–9.

164. Littorin M, Hou S, Broberg K, et al. Influence of polymorphic metabolic enzymes on biotransformation and effects of diphenylmethane diisocyanate. Int Arch Occup Environ Health 2008;81:429–41.

165. Wisnewski AV, Liu Q, Liu J, et al. Glutathione protects human airway proteins and epithelial cells from isocyanates. Clin Exp Allergy 2005;35:352–7.

166. Kim SH, Cho BY, Park CS, et al. Alpha-T-catenin (CTNNA3) gene was identified as a risk variant for toluene diisocyanate-induced asthma by genome-wide association analysis. Clin Exp Allergy 2009;39:203–12.

Clinical Assessment of Occupational Asthma and its Differential Diagnosis

André Cartier, MD[a],*, Joaquin Sastre, MD, PhD[b]

KEYWORDS

- Occupational asthma • Peak expiratory flow monitoring
- Specific inhalation challenges • Diagnosis • Skin tests
- Sputum induction • Questionnaire

Asthma is the most frequent respiratory disease, affecting up to 8% of adult working populations. Population-based studies have estimated that the proportion of adult-onset asthma caused by occupational exposures ranges from 5% to 10% in Europe, 10% to 23% in the United States, to 17% to 29% in Finland. The proportion of persons with asthma who experience worsening symptoms caused by work activities or environments is not well known, ranging between 16% and 31%, depending on the study design and population studied.[1]

Work-related asthma refers to asthma that is attributable to, or is worsened by, environmental exposures in the workplace. It can be categorized into occupational asthma (OA) and work-exacerbated asthma (WEA). Several definitions have been given to both terms.[1–3] OA is defined as asthma caused by sources and conditions attributable to a particular occupational environment and not to stimuli encountered outside the workplace.[4] Two types of OA are distinguished based on their appearance after a latency period or not. The most frequent type, which is usually quoted as OA, appears after a latency period leading to sensitization, either allergic or immunoglobulin E (IgE)-mediated like most high- and certain low-molecular-weight agents or through unknown mechanisms. The other type does not require a latency period and includes irritant-induced asthma or reactive dysfunction syndrome, which may occur after single or multiple exposures to high concentrations of nonspecific irritants.[5,6] WEA, or work-aggravated asthma, can be defined as the worsening of preexisting or coincident (new-onset) asthma by workplace exposures.

[a] Hôpital du Sacré-Cœur de Montréal, 5400 Boul Gouin Ouest, Montréal, QC, Canada, H4J 1C5
[b] Allergy Department, Fundación Jiménez Díaz, Avda. Reyes Católicos, 2, 28040, Madrid, Spain
* Corresponding author.
E-mail address: andre.cartier@umontreal.ca

Immunol Allergy Clin N Am 31 (2011) 717–728
doi:10.1016/j.iac.2011.07.005   immunology.theclinics.com
0889-8561/11/$ – see front matter © 2011 Elsevier Inc. All rights reserved.

The purpose of the review is to outline the clinical assessment and differential diagnosis of sensitizer-induced OA.

HOW TO MAKE THE DIAGNOSIS OF OA?

The diagnosis of OA relies on the objective evidence that asthma is triggered by work exposure; it needs to be distinguished from WEA and other conditions that may mimic asthma at work.

The different steps involved in the investigation of work-related asthma are history; pulmonary function tests; immunologic tests; combined results of serial peak expiratory flow (PEF) monitoring, nonallergic bronchial responsiveness (NABR), and sputum induction; and specific bronchial challenges. Although specific inhalation challenges (SIC) are considered the diagnostic reference standard, all steps involved in the investigation have their own value and contribute to establishing the diagnosis. Combining the various elements strengthens the likelihood of a proper diagnosis.

History

The classical history of OA is one of a worker whose asthma is worse at work, improving over weekends or holidays. However, even workers without work-related asthma regularly report improvement of asthma during weekends and holidays (41% and 54% of cases, respectively).[7] Furthermore, this pattern is often absent because symptoms are also usually present outside the workplace and triggered by exposure to irritants, such as cold air, fumes, or exercise. The concomitant occurrence of rhinoconjunctivitis at work, especially in a worker exposed to high-molecular-weight chemicals who develops asthma, is surely suggestive of OA.[8] Symptoms may develop after latency periods of only a few weeks or several years; the duration of exposure tends to be shorter for low-molecular-weight chemicals.[9] A previous history of asthma does not exclude the diagnosis of OA.

Physicians evaluating workers with possible OA should inquire about exposure to potential sensitizers and irritants, either directly or indirectly. Work that generates dust, such as the use of abrasive materials, or devices and work locations in which there are strong odors or where combustion or chemical reactions are taking place are often problematic because they may trigger asthma symptoms through irritant or sensitizing mechanisms. Material safety data sheets may be useful to document the nature of exposure to any sensitizing or irritant agents; but they are not always consistent in their format and content and may not identify sensitizing substances as such, particularly if present at low concentrations in the product or its ingredients (ie, <1%).[10]

Even if the history is essential to make a diagnosis of asthma, it is often misleading. Indeed, several studies have shown that asthma is overdiagnosed in the general population because of the lack of objective confirmation of the diagnosis. Aaron and colleagues[11] showed that among 492 subjects with physician-diagnosed asthma, nearly one-third did not have asthma when objectively assessed after medication withdrawal and proper follow-up. In occupational settings, the authors have previously shown that a diagnosis of OA based on clinical history has a positive predictive value of only 63%[12]; among those with a very likely or likely diagnosis of OA, 13.5% had even no objective evidence of asthma. Furthermore, among 169 subjects referred for respiratory symptoms suggestive of work-related asthma, Chiry and colleagues[13] have shown that 69 (40.8%) had no objective evidence of asthma, although the type and severity of their respiratory symptoms were similar to those reported by subjects with confirmed asthma except for wheezing, which was more frequent in the latter group.

Therefore, a suggestive history, even in the presence of a know sensitizer, is not enough to confirm the diagnosis of asthma or of OA. The diagnosis needs to be confirmed objectively.

Confirming the Diagnosis of Asthma

The diagnosis of asthma is based on history and objective evidence of reversible airflow obstruction or increased NABR[14,15] as determined by methacholine inhalation challenges with determination of the provocative concentration of methacholine inducing a 20% fall in forced expiratory volume in one second (FEV1) or PC20M. Unfortunately, this is often neglected, as shown by a study of Curwick and colleagues[16] whereby less than half of the individuals who had filed a claim for work-related asthma had received an objective evaluation of pulmonary function, whereas only 27% had tests for reversible airflow limitation.

Although documentation of reversible airflow limitation confirms the diagnosis of asthma, most workers investigated for OA have normal spirometry when seen in the clinic. Furthermore, preshift and postshift monitoring of FEV1 has not proven sensitive or specific enough to be a useful tool in the evaluation of OA.[17]

Even if increased NABR is the hallmark of asthma, its presence does not alone establish the diagnosis of OA. It may suggest that patients have OA, common asthma, or other conditions that are associated with increased NABR, such as allergic rhinitis or chronic obstructive lung disease. There is a need for further confirmation of work-related asthma. The absence of increased NABR assessed shortly (minutes, hours) after a work shift in a worker with symptoms virtually excludes OA.[18] In rare instances, however, specific inhalation challenges have been positive in workers without increased NABR. Even in workers with confirmed OA, NABR may normalize after several days (a weekend may be enough[19]) or weeks to months away from work. Subsequent return to work or even exposure via a specific inhalation test may be then restore increased NABR in the asthmatic range.[20,21]

Skin Tests and Serology

The presence of immediate skin test reactivity or increased serum-specific IgE or IgG antibodies may reflect sensitization or exposure to a suspect agent but do not prove target organ sensitization (the bronchi in this instance). Allergy tests can, however, be quite useful in supporting the diagnosis and may help to identify which of the multiple suspect agents may be relevant.

With most high-molecular-weight agents for which test extracts are commercially available, such as cereals, negative skin prick tests cannot entirely exclude the diagnosis of OA but make it very unlikely. Indeed, the worker may still be sensitized to another agent found in the workplace or to another component of the offending material. Conversely, a positive skin test confirms IgE-mediated sensitization but does not confirm the OA because its positive predictive value is low. With most low-molecular-weight chemicals, skin test antigens or serum-specific IgE or IgG immunoassays are either not available commercially or lack established test validity to refute or to make a diagnosis of OA. Other in vitro tests, such as basophil histamine release or assay of monocyte chemoattractant protein-1 by peripheral blood mononuclear cells,[22] may offer higher sensitivity or specificity, but again they do not alone confirm the diagnosis of OA.

Although specific inhalation challenges are considered the reference test, they are not always available, and combining various tests increases the likelihood of a correct diagnosis. In the case of high-molecular-weight agents, combining a history highly suggestive of OA with a positive methacholine challenge and a positive skin test to a high-molecular-weight agent gives a post-test probability of greater than 90% of the disease. On the other hand, negative combined test results do not seem to provide clinicians with a sufficient predictive value to rule out OA.[23]

Monitoring of PEF, NABR, and Sputum at Work and off Work

The availability of portable, inexpensive devices has allowed physicians to monitor PEF at work and off work.[24–27] This monitoring can be coupled with the monitoring of nonallergic bronchial responsiveness and the counting of inflammatory cells in induced sputum.[28] When compared with specific inhalation challenges as the reference, PEF monitoring has a sensitivity of around 64% and a specificity of 77%, with visual analysis being the best way to evaluate changes in PEF. A computer-based system analysis of PEF has been developed by Gannon and colleagues and validated as a useful tool to assess work-related changes in PEF.[29–31]

Ideally, PEF should be measured every 2 hours for at least 2 weeks at work and off work.[32] Moore and colleagues have shown that when PEF are measured at least 8 times per day, the area between the curves score can shorten the period of required monitoring to at least 8 working days and 3 days off work, with a sensitivity of 68% and a specificity of 91%[33]; this may improve worker compliance with the collection of PEF data. In certain situations, particularly when asthma is severe or when the nature of the offending agent is unknown or intermittent, interpretation of the monitoring data may be difficult.[34] Patients should be asked to take rescue beta-2 agonists on demand only but should continue their inhaled steroids regularly. Indeed, reduction of inhaled steroids on return to work may be associated with deterioration of asthma and decrease in PEF, which may be mistaken as diagnostic of OA (or a false positive test). During collection of PEFs, long-acting beta-2 agonists and leukotrienes antagonists should be avoided, but continuation of theophylline at the same dosage is permitted. In patients with severe asthma, it may be necessary to initially withdraw them from work until asthma control has been achieved and before returning back to work on minimal controller therapy; subsequent deterioration of asthma may then imply that asthma is caused by work.

The poor sensitivity or specificity of PEF monitoring in certain patients compared with specific bronchial challenges can be related to several factors. On one hand, PEF may greatly underestimate or overestimate changes in airway caliber as assessed by FEV1.[35–37] On the other hand, they are effort dependent and, thus, require the cooperation of the worker, which is not always obtained because of the fear of losing his or her job or malingering to gain compensation benefits.[38,39]

The combination of NABR monitoring and PEF monitoring at work and off work is now frequently used in the investigation of OA. Indeed, although exposure to irritants does not induce marked and prolonged changes in NABR, OA may be associated with significant and often long-lasting changes in NABR. When significant changes in PEF are associated with parallel changes in NABR, the diagnosis of OA is highly probable. If the monitoring of PEF and NABR are discordant, further investigations should be completed, such as specific bronchial challenges in the workplace or in the laboratory. Finally, when monitoring of PEF and NABR show no evidence of asthma in symptomatic patients actively exposed to suspect causative agents at work, the diagnosis of OA can be excluded.

However, Chiry and colleagues[40] showed that the interpretation of PEF alone cannot accurately distinguish WEA from OA, even if the magnitude of PEF variability at work is greater in patients with OA. Girard and colleagues[28] showed that sputum eosinophils may increase following return to work in patients with OA compared with those with WEA. The authors, therefore, routinely use a combination of PEF,

NABR, and sputum monitoring in the evaluation of work-related asthma. Discrepant or ambiguous results between any of these tests are resolved by investigation with specific inhalation challenge studies.

Finally, although monitoring of PEF and NABR (± sputum counts) are useful tools, they are time consuming, require patient collaboration, and uncontrolled work exposure may be hazardous in workers reporting severe asthma at work. Exposure may not be titrated as easily as during a controlled challenge conducted in the laboratory. Testing in the workplace is particularly useful as a screening procedure when the worker is exposed to several sensitizers or when the offending agent is unknown.

Specific Inhalation Challenges

These tests are still considered the reference test to confirm the diagnosis of OA.[17,41] Originally done in the laboratory and aiming to mimic work exposure, these are now frequently done in the workplace.

SIC are safe when performed under the close supervision of an expert physician and by trained personnel and are, thus, limited to specialized centers. Although there is no standardized protocol, the methodology is well developed.[42] Resuscitative measures should be readily available. Drugs should be withheld before specific bronchial challenges according to standard recommendations.[42] When performed in the laboratory, the exposure chambers should be well ventilated and enclosed to minimize exposure to the personnel. The tests can be performed on an outpatient basis. Most challenges are done in an open fashion, with patients knowing the nature of the exposure.

Whereas FEV1 is the standard parameter used to assess changes in airway caliber, PEF are not reliable enough, particularly during the early asthmatic response because they may underestimate or overestimate changes.[35] In all cases, spirometry should be monitored on a control day to ensure the stability of airway caliber at regular intervals for at least 8 hours. At the end of the control day, the authors routinely do a methacholine challenge test followed by sputum induction.

When performed in the laboratory, specific bronchial challenges can be done in several ways, depending on the nature of the agent (ie, powder, aerosol, liquid, or gas). With powders, like flour or red cedar, patients may be exposed to a fine dust that mimics work exposure by pouring the dust from one tray to another. Using a dust generator allows proper monitoring, regulation of exposure, generation of dose-response curves, and reduces the risks of severe bronchospasm or irritant reactions.[43] The agent may be diluted initially with an inert agent, such as lactose, to avoid severe reactions. Alternatively, the worker may be exposed to an aerosol of a crude extract. Exposure to nonpowder agents is usually done by reproducing the work environment (eg, by having the worker breath over a bottle of methacrylate glue). Isocyanates and other gases can be generated in their gaseous or aerosol form in a closed-circuit generating chamber or a whole-body exposure chamber. Whenever possible, the level of exposure should be continuously monitored to avoid high exposure and, therefore, irritant reactions.

Baseline spirometry on each exposure day should be reproducible (ie, ≤10% of the control day). The exposure should be progressive (eg, 1 breath, 10–15 seconds, 1 minute, 2 minutes, 5 minutes, and so forth). The maximal duration of exposure is usually 2 hours. The dose may be conveniently increased sequentially by serial increases of the exposure period or increasing the concentration of the agent. If there is no significant variation in FEV1 on the last exposure day, NABR and sputum induction should be reassessed at the end of that day. If there is no significant change in FEV1 from baseline but the PC20M is significantly lower (ie, >3.2-fold change in PC20M) or if there is a significant increase in sputum eosinophils (ie, increase of

2.2% in eosinophil count), the same exposure level is repeated on the next day for up to 4 hours because the test may then be positive.[44,45]

Tests in the workplace are now done more frequently, especially when the relevant agent at work is unknown or when there are several potential sensitizing agents. They are also done stepwise because patients may experience a significant decrease in FEV1. Spirometry is followed in the same way throughout the day. Exposure to the offending agent is, however, less well controlled and monitored than in the laboratory and it may be difficult to ensure that patients are really exposed to the relevant agent at work. This may be, however, the only way to confirm the diagnosis of OA especially in cases whereby the nature of the offending agent is unknown.

A significant reaction is defined as a 20% decrease in FEV1 from the preexposure baseline FEV1. Typical patterns of bronchial reactions have been described.[46] Immediate asthmatic reactions are maximal between 10 and 30 minutes after exposure with complete recovery within 1 to 2 hours; although usually readily reversible by inhaled beta-2 agonists, they are actually the most dangerous because they can be severe and unpredictable, particularly in patients for whom skin tests with the suspecting agent are not possible, stressing the importance of progressive exposure. Late asthmatic reactions develop slowly and progressively either 1 to 2 hours (early late) or 4 to 8 hours (late) after exposure. If late responses are accompanied by fever and general malaise, extrinsic alveolitis should be considered. Dual reactions are a combination of early and late.

Atypical patterns[46] have also been described with isocyanates and other low- or high-molecular-weight chemicals and include (1) the progressive type (starting within minutes after end of exposure and progressing over the next 7–8 hours); (2) the square-waved reaction (with no recovery between the immediate and late components of the reaction); and finally (3) the prolonged immediate type with slow recovery. Low-molecular-weight chemicals are more often associated with atypical patterns as compared with high-molecular-weight proteins.

Irritant reactions are not well characterized, but decreases in FEV1 that recover rapidly within 10 or 20 minutes are suggestive of an irritant pattern. It may be impossible to interpret results of specific bronchial challenges in patients with exaggerated daily variability in FEV1, which stresses the importance of an adequate control day.

A positive test confirms the diagnosis of OA, whereas a negative test in the workplace, or in the laboratory, does not absolutely rule out the diagnosis of OA in a worker who has not been exposed to work for several months because he may have become desensitized. This point is particularly true if there is a change in PC20M following a negative response to specific inhalation challenges. Such a worker should return to work for serial monitoring of PEF and bronchial responsiveness for at least a few weeks before excluding the diagnosis. False negative challenges in the laboratory may also be caused by exposure to the wrong agent or the inadvertent administration of a forbidden drug (eg, inhaled beta-2 agonist) before the test. However, if patients experience their usual symptoms during the challenge procedure without any spirometric changes, these tests are conclusive and exclude the diagnosis of OA.

WHAT IS CONSIDERED IN THE DIFFERENTIAL DIAGNOSIS OF OA?

Several clinical entities can be confused with OA and, therefore, must be considered in its differential diagnosis, especially those that mimic asthma (**Box 1**). Furthermore, it must be kept in mind that any entity simulating asthma may coexist with OA.

WEA refers to asthma triggered by various work-related factors (eg, aeroallergens, irritants, or exercise) in workers who are known to have preexisting or coincident

---

Box 1
Differential diagnosis of OA

Work-exacerbated asthma

Irritant-induced asthma

Chronic obstructive pulmonary disease

Occupational and nonoccupational rhinitis

Hyperventilation syndrome and panic attacks

Bronchiolitis

Hypersensitivity pneumonitis

Eosinophilic bronchitis

Vocal cord dysfunction and irritable larynx syndrome

Multiple chemical sensitivity syndrome

(new-onset) asthma.[27] The frequency of WEA varies from 36% to 58% of all work-related asthma cases[1] depending on the asthma criteria used (eg, an asthma questionnaire or physician diagnosis). On average, persons presenting with WEA are older and tend to be nonwhite, have a low income level, a more severe form of the disease, and more difficult access to respiratory care than other adults with asthma.[47] Definitive diagnosis of WEA should be based on objective indicators of asthma exacerbation related to the work environment, such as the greater use of asthma medication, increased frequency of physician or hospital visits, or worsened pulmonary function (as determined by PEFR or spirometry or nonspecific bronchial hyperresponsiveness). SIC may be performed to rule out the possibility of sensitization to a suspected allergen, thus, making SIC a crucial component of evaluation for WEA.[1]

Chronic obstructive pulmonary disease should be considered in patients experiencing dyspnea at work. A history of smoking, chronic cough and phlegm, and irreversible airways obstruction will help to make the diagnosis.

Hyperventilation syndrome is frequently misdiagnosed as asthma.[12,48] It is characterized by a variety of somatic symptoms induced by physiologically inappropriate hyperventilation and usually reproduced in whole or in part by voluntary hyperventilation. Panic attacks, which are also associated with hyperventilation syndrome, may also develop after acute irritant exposures.

Cough associated with rhinitis, either occupational or not, may mimic symptoms of asthma and should be considered in the investigation of workers with suspected OA. Other causes of cough can also mimic asthma as reviewed by Tarlo and colleagues.[49]

The term bronchiolitis applies to various diseases involving inflammation of the bronchioles, small airways, and occasionally of the alveoli, leading to airflow obstruction. The symptoms will depend on the underlying disease, although most patients will present with cough, dyspnea, tightness of the chest, and occasionally expectoration or wheezing.[50] Workers in popcorn factories can develop both occupational asthma[51] and bronchiolitis,[52] the latter caused by exposure to diacetyl. A lymphocytic bronchiolitis has also been described in workers employed in the nylon industry.[53]

Some of the agents that cause OA, such as diisocyanates and fungal spores, can also cause hypersensitivity pneumonitis (HP). Although uncommonly, HP can be associated with wheezing, airway hyperresponsiveness, and a normal chest radiograph.[54,55] The diagnosis of HP is based on the recurrence of systemic symptoms occurring 4 to 8 hours after exposure to a known offending antigen, weight loss, inspiratory crackles observed on physical examination, positive precipitating antibodies to the offending antigen, compatible results in high-resolution computed tomography scan and bronchoalveolar lavage, and reduced lung diffusion capacity with or without volume restriction.

Eosinophilic bronchitis causes chronic cough with phlegm, dyspnea, and, on rare occasions, wheezing. It is characterized by increased eosinophils in sputum (>3%) in the absence of increased NABR.[56] Cases of eosinophilic bronchitis have been described as being associated with exposure to certain workplace-related substances. Occupational eosinophilic bronchitis is characterized by the presence of isolated chronic cough (lasting more than 3 weeks) that worsens at work; sputum eosinophilia (>3% in sputum); increase in sputum eosinophils related to exposure to the offending agent (either at work or after SIC); normal spirometric parameters that are not significantly affected by exposure to the offending agent; absence of bronchial hyperresponsiveness to methacholine and adenosine both at work and away from work; and when other causes of chronic cough are ruled out.[57] This entity reinforces the importance of examining induced sputum as part of the diagnostic algorithm for individuals who complain of asthmalike symptoms in the workplace.[58]

Vocal cord dysfunction (VCD) is characterized by paradoxic vocal cord adduction during inhalation. This anomalous adduction causes airflow to be obstructed and may be manifested as dysphonia, stridor, wheezing, tightness of the chest, dyspnea, or cough. Thus, it may mimic asthma and should always be considered in the differential diagnosis of patients with asthmalike symptoms that fail to respond to conventional asthma therapy. Although this condition has been associated with psychiatric disorders, it has also been linked to certain types of workplace exposure varying from irritants to specific agents, and can be an important cause of work-associated respiratory symptoms.[59–61] However, loss of voice occurring in cases of OA induced by high-molecular-weight agents has been significantly negatively associated with the presence of OA.[62] VCD is suspected on spirometry results with the flattening of the inspiratory limb of the maximum flow-volume loop, with or without a decrease in FEV1. To confirm the diagnosis, fiberoptic rhinolaryngoscopy is performed at a time when symptoms are present. Recently, Hoy and colleagues,[63] have reported that occupational exposures may initiate or trigger recurrent hyperkinetic laryngeal symptoms, predominantly episodic dyspnea, dysphonia, cough, and sensation of tension in the throat. The investigators have coined this work-associated irritable larynx syndrome (WILS). Patients experiencing WILS were more likely to be women and more frequently reported symptoms of gastroesophageal reflux. The most common triggers of workplace symptoms in the WILS group were odors, fumes, perfumes, and cleaning agents. Fourteen of 30 patients with WILS identified a specific precipitating event at the workplace at the time of the onset of their symptoms, and 5 of these patients presented to an emergency department within 24 hours of the event.

Multiple chemical sensitivity syndrome or idiopathic environmental intolerance is a condition acquired following a documented toxic exposure and is usually characterized by recurrent symptoms that affect multiple organ systems.[64] Exposure-related symptoms associated with self-reported multiple chemical sensitivities can be divided into nonspecific complaints of the central nervous system (main characteristic) and functional disturbances in other organ systems (optional complaints). Patients may, thus, report cough, dyspnea, tightness of the chest, and retrosternal chest pain during exposures. The condition commonly leads to a substantial reduction in patient quality of life, and a significant overlap is seen with fibromyalgia. Physical examination is usually normal, as are the various complementary tests, including lung function tests and measure of NABR.

SUMMARY

Although it is difficult to distinguish WEA from OA, a combination of tools will help the clinician to come to a proper diagnosis. Other conditions mimicking asthma should also be considered. Objective confirmation of asthma and work-related asthma is essential because history is neither sensitive nor specific enough to come to a proper diagnosis. SIC performed in the workplace or laboratory is still considered the reference standard to confirm the diagnosis.

REFERENCES

1. Lemière C. Occupational and work-exacerbated asthma: similarities and differences. Expert Rev Respir Med 2007;1(1):43–9.
2. Vandenplas O, Malo JL. Definitions and types of work-related asthma: a nosological approach. Eur Respir J 2003;21(4):706–12.
3. Wagner GR, Henneberger PK. Asthma exacerbated at work. In: Bernstein IL, Chan-Yeung M, Malo JL, et al, editors. Asthma in the workplace and related conditions. New York: Taylor & Francis Group; 2006. p. 631–40.
4. Bernstein IL, Bernstein DI, Chan-Yeung M, et al. Definition and classification of asthma in the workplace. In: Bernstein IL, Chan-Yeung M, Malo JL, editors. Asthma in the workplace and related conditions. New York: Taylor & Francis Group; 2006. p. 1–8.
5. Brooks SM, Weiss MA, Bernstein IL. Reactive airways dysfunction syndrome (RADS). Persistent asthma syndrome after high level irritant exposures. Chest 1985;88(3):376–84.
6. Brooks SM, Bernstein IL. Reactive airways dysfunction syndrome or irritant-induced asthma. In: Bernstein IL, Chan-Yeung M, Malo JL, et al, editors. Asthma in the workplace. New York: Marcel Decker Inc; 1993. p. 533–49.
7. Tarlo SM, Liss G, Corey P, et al. A workers compensation claim population for occupational asthma - comparison of subgroups. Chest 1995;107(3):634–41.
8. Malo JL, Lemière C, Desjardins A, et al. Prevalence and intensity of rhinoconjunctivitis in subjects with occupational asthma. Eur Respir J 1997;10(7):1513–5.
9. Malo JL, Ghezzo H, D'Aquino C, et al. Natural history of occupational asthma: relevance of type of agent and other factors in the rate of development of symptoms in affected subjects. J Allergy Clin Immunol 1992;90:937–44.
10. Bernstein JA. Material safety data sheets: are they reliable in identifying human hazards? J Allergy Clin Immunol 2002;110(1):35–8.
11. Aaron SD, Vandemheen KL, Boulet LP, et al. Overdiagnosis of asthma in obese and nonobese adults. Can Med Assoc J 2008;179(11):1121–31.
12. Malo JL, Ghezzo H, L'Archeveque J, et al. Is the clinical history a satisfactory means of diagnosing occupational asthma? Am Rev Respir Dis 1991;143:528–32.
13. Chiry S, Boulet LP, Lepage J, et al. Frequency of work-related respiratory symptoms in workers without asthma. Am J Ind Med 2009;52(6):447–54.
14. Lougheed MD, Lemière C, Dell SD, et al. Canadian Thoracic Society Asthma Management Continuum - 2010 Consensus Summary for children six years of age and over, and adults. Can Respir J 2010;17(1):15–24.
15. Global initiative for asthma. Global strategy of asthma management and prevention. Revised 2009. Available at: http://www.ginasthma.org. Accessed August 25, 2011.
16. Curwick CC, Bonauto DK, Adams DA. Use of objective testing in the diagnosis of work-related asthma by physician specialty. Ann Allergy Asthma Immunol 2006; 97(4):546–50.

17. Nicholson PJ, Cullinan P, Taylor AJ, et al. Evidence based guidelines for the prevention, identification, and management of occupational asthma. Occup Environ Med 2005;62(5):290–9.

18. Baur X, Huber H, Degens PO, et al. Relation between occupational asthma case history, bronchial methacholine challenge, and specific challenge test in patients with suspected occupational asthma. Am J Ind Med 1998;33(2):114–22.

19. Cockcroft DW, Mink JT. Isocyanate-induced asthma in an automobile spray painter. Can Med Assoc J 1979;121(5):602–4.

20. Hargreave FE, Ramsdale EH, Pugsley SO. Occupational asthma without bronchial hyperresponsiveness. Am Rev Respir Dis 1984;130:513–5.

21. Lemière C, Cartier A, Dolovich J, et al. Outcome of specific bronchial responsiveness to occupational agents after removal from exposure. Am J Respir Crit Care Med 1996;154(2 Pt 1):329–33.

22. Bernstein DI, Cartier A, Côté J, et al. Diisocyanate antigen-stimulated monocyte chemoattractant protein-1 synthesis has greater test efficiency than specific antibodies for identification of diisocyanate asthma. Am J Respir Crit Care Med 2002; 166(4):445–50.

23. Beach J, Russell K, Blitz S, et al. A systematic review of the diagnosis of occupational asthma. Chest 2007;131(2):569–78.

24. Moscato G, Godnic-Cvar J, Maestrelli P, et al. Statement on self-monitoring of peak expiratory flows in the investigation of occupational asthma. Subcommittee on Occupational Allergy of the European Academy of Allergology and Clinical Immunology. American Academy of Allergy and Clinical Immunology. European Respiratory Society. American College of Allergy, Asthma and Immunology. Eur Respir J 1995;8(9):1605–10.

25. Bright P, Burge PS. Occupational lung disease. 8. The diagnosis of occupational asthma from serial measurements of lung function at and away from work. Thorax 1996;51(8):857–63.

26. Beach J, Rowe BH, Blitz S, et al. Evidence Report/Technology Assessment No. 129. Diagnosis and management of work-related asthma. Rockville (MD): Agency for Healthcare Research and Quality; 2005.

27. Tarlo SM, Balmes J, Balkissoon R, et al. Diagnosis and management of work-related asthma: American College of Chest Physicians Consensus Statement. Chest 2008;134(Suppl 3):1S–41S.

28. Girard F, Chaboillez S, Cartier A, et al. An effective strategy for diagnosing occupational asthma: use of induced sputum. Am J Respir Crit Care Med 2004;170(8): 845–50.

29. Gannon PFG, Newton DT, Belcher J, et al. Development of OASYS-2-a system for the analysis of serial measurement of peak expiratory flow in workers with suspected occupational asthma. Thorax 1996;51(5):484–9.

30. Bright P, Newton DT, Gannon PF, et al. OASYS-3: improved analysis of serial peak expiratory flow in suspected occupational asthma. Monaldi Arch Chest Dis 2001; 56(3):281–8.

31. Baldwin DR, Gannon P, Bright P, et al. Interpretation of occupational peak flow records: level of agreement between expert clinicians and Oasys-2. Thorax 2002;57(10):860–4.

32. Malo JL, Côté J, Cartier A, et al. How many times per day should peak expiratory flow rates be assessed when investigating occupational asthma? Thorax 1993; 48(12):1211–7.

33. Moore VC, Jaakkola MS, Burge CB, et al. PEF analysis requiring shorter records for occupational asthma diagnosis. Occup Med (Lond) 2009;59(6):413–7.

34. Perrin B, Lagier F, L'Archeveque J, et al. Occupational asthma: validity of monitoring of peak expiratory flow rates and non-allergic bronchial responsiveness as compared to specific inhalation challenge. Eur Respir J 1992;5:40–8.
35. Bérubé D, Cartier A, L'Archeveque J, et al. Comparison of peak expiratory flow rate and FEV1 in assessing bronchomotor tone after challenges with occupational sensitizers. Chest 1991;99:831–6.
36. Gautrin D, D'Aquino LC, Gagnon G, et al. Comparison between peak expiratory flow rates (PEFR) and FEV_1 in the monitoring of asthmatic subjects at the outpatient clinic. Chest 1994;106:1419–26.
37. Moscato G, Dellabianca A, Paggiaro P, et al. Peak expiratory flow monitoring and airway response to specific bronchial provocation tests in asthmatics. Monaldi Arch Chest Dis 1993;48:23–8.
38. Malo JL, Trudeau C, Ghezzo H, et al. Do subjects investigated for occupational asthma through serial peak expiratory flow measurements falsify their results. J Allergy Clin Immunol 1995;96(5 Part 1):601–7.
39. Quirce S, Contreras G, Dybuncio A, et al. Peak expiratory flow monitoring is not a reliable method for establishing the diagnosis of occupational asthma. Am J Respir Crit Care Med 1995;152(3):1100–2.
40. Chiry S, Cartier A, Malo JL, et al. Comparison of peak expiratory flow variability between workers with work-exacerbated asthma and occupational asthma. Chest 2007;132(2):483–8.
41. Newman Taylor AJ, Cullinan P, Burge PS, et al. BOHRF guidelines for occupational asthma. Thorax 2005;60(5):364–6.
42. Cartier A, Bernstein IL, Burge PS, et al. Guidelines for bronchoprovocation on the investigation of occupational asthma. Report of the Subcommittee on Bronchoprovocation for Occupational Asthma. J Allergy Clin Immunol 1989;84(5 Pt 2): 823–9.
43. Cloutier Y, Lagier F, Cartier A, et al. Validation of an exposure system to particles for the diagnosis of occupational asthma. Chest 1992;102:402–7.
44. Vandenplas O, Delwiche JP, Jamart J, et al. Increase in non-specific bronchial hyperresponsiveness as an early marker of bronchial response to occupational agents during specific inhalation challenges. Thorax 1996;51(5):472–8.
45. Vandenplas O, D'Alpaos V, Heymans J, et al. Sputum eosinophilia: an early marker of bronchial response to occupational agents. Allergy 2009;64(5):754–61.
46. Perrin B, Cartier A, Ghezzo H, et al. Reassessment of the temporal patterns of bronchial obstruction after exposure to occupational sensitizing agents. J Allergy Clin Immunol 1991;87:630–9.
47. Henneberger PK. Work-exacerbated asthma. Curr Opin Allergy Clin Immunol 2007;7(2):146–51.
48. Thomas M, McKinley RK, Freeman E, et al. Prevalence of dysfunctional breathing in patients treated for asthma in primary care: cross sectional survey. BMJ 2001; 322(7294):1098–100.
49. Tarlo SM. Cough: occupational and environmental considerations: ACCP evidence-based clinical practice guidelines. Chest 2006;129(Suppl 1): 186S–96S.
50. Ryu JH, Myers JL, Swensen SJ. Bronchiolar disorders. Am J Respir Crit Care Med 2003;168(11):1277–92.
51. Sahakian N, Kullman G, Lynch D, et al. Asthma arising in flavoring-exposed food production workers. Int J Occup Med Environ Health 2008;21(2):173–7.
52. Kreiss K, Gomaa A, Kullman G, et al. Clinical bronchiolitis obliterans in workers at a microwave-popcorn plant. N Engl J Med 2002;347(5):330–8.

53. Boag AH, Colby TV, Fraire AE, et al. The pathology of interstitial lung disease in nylon flock workers. Am J Surg Pathol 1999;23(12):1539–45.

54. Lacasse Y, Selman M, Costabel U, et al. Clinical diagnosis of hypersensitivity pneumonitis. Am J Respir Crit Care Med 2003;168(8):952–8.

55. Fink JN, Ortega HG, Reynolds HY, et al. Needs and opportunities for research in hypersensitivity pneumonitis. Am J Respir Crit Care Med 2005;171(7):792–8.

56. Brightling CE. Chronic cough due to nonasthmatic eosinophilic bronchitis: ACCP evidence-based clinical practice guidelines. Chest 2006;129(Suppl 1): 116S–21S.

57. Quirce S. Eosinophilic bronchitis in the workplace. Curr Opin Allergy Clin Immunol 2004;4(2):87–91.

58. Quirce S, Lemière C, De BF, et al. Noninvasive methods for assessment of airway inflammation in occupational settings. Allergy 2010;65(4):445–58.

59. Perkner JJ, Fennelly KP, Balkissoon R, et al. Irritant-associated vocal cord dysfunction. J Occup Environ Med 1998;40(2):136–43.

60. Galdi E, Perfetti L, Pagella F, et al. Irritant vocal cord dysfunction at first misdiagnosed as reactive airway dysfunction syndrome. Scand J Work Environ Health 2005;31(3):224–6.

61. Tonini S, Dellabianca A, Costa C, et al. Irritant vocal cord dysfunction and occupational bronchial asthma: differential diagnosis in a health care worker. Int J Occup Med Environ Health 2009;22(4):401–6.

62. Vandenplas O, Ghezzo H, Munoz X, et al. What are the questionnaire items most useful in identifying subjects with occupational asthma? Eur Respir J 2005;26(6): 1056–63.

63. Hoy RF, Ribeiro M, Anderson J, et al. Work-associated irritable larynx syndrome. Occup Med (Lond) 2010;60(7):546–51.

64. Cullen MR. The worker with multiple chemical sensitivities: an overview. Occup Med 1987;2(4):655–61.

Work-Related Asthma: A Case-Based Approach to Management

Karin A. Pacheco, MD, MSPH[a], Susan M. Tarlo, MB BS, FRCP(C)[b],*

KEYWORDS

- Occupational asthma • Work-exacerbated asthma
- Work-aggravated asthma • Work-related asthma
- Management

The pharmacologic treatment of work-related asthma is the same as for nonoccupational asthma, following the National Heart, Lung, and Blood Institute (NHLBI)[1] or Global Initiative on Asthma (GINA) guidelines.[2] However, additional concerns related to managing workplace exposures, job and task modifications, and medicolegal aspects make work-related asthma more complicated to manage.[3] This article focuses mainly on those issues that are more specific to work-related asthma, to provide insight and direction as to how to manage these additional, more problematic aspects. Finally, it discusses levels and methods of prevention as the best management for occupationally induced or exacerbated asthma. Each category of work-related asthma—occupational asthma (OA) and work-exacerbated asthma (WEA)—begins with a case vignette illustrating management issues specific to that type of asthma.

HIGH-MOLECULAR-WEIGHT SENSITIZER-INDUCED ASTHMA
Case Example

A 30-year-old woman without a past history of asthma or allergies worked as a dental assistant for the past 10 years. Three years ago she developed red, raised, itchy welts

Disclosures: Dr Susan Tarlo has received peer-reviewed research grant funding from the Ontario Workplace Safety and Insurance Board and from WorkSafeBC and the Workers' Compensation Board of Newfoundland and Labrador for studies on work-related asthma.
Disclosure: Dr Karin Pacheco has received research funding from the National Institute of Allergy and Infectious Diseases, National Institutes of Health for studies on occupational asthma.

[a] Department of Medicine, National Jewish Health, Colorado School of Public Health, University of Colorado, CO, USA
[b] Department of Medicine, University of Toronto, and Dalla Lana School of Public Health, Toronto Western Hospital, EW7-449, 399 Bathurst Street, Toronto, Ontario, M5T 2S8, Canada
* Corresponding author.
E-mail address: susan.tarlo@utoronto.ca

on her arms, anterior chest, and neck that usually appeared at work but were absent on vacations. They typically occurred 2 to 3 times a week, lasting 30 to 60 minutes, and resolved when she took oral antihistamines. Over the past year, she developed episodic cough, shortness of breath, and chest tightness, sometimes at work and sometimes in the evening after work. Her hives have not resolved after switching to nitrile gloves, and coworkers also only use nitrile gloves.

The patient's job entails a variety of different tasks and some exposures to potentially sensitizing materials. She makes impressions for bleach trays using an alginate impression material (cell-wall constituents of brown algae). She performs in-office bleaching using concentrated hydrogen peroxide, and also applies a phosphoric acid etching solution to each tooth before applying a resin base for a crown. She applies restorative composites of dimethacrylates and bisphenol A, and much of her time is spent cementing crowns in place using a two-part paste of ethyl and dimethacrylates, bisphenol A, and benzoyl peroxide. She also assists with minor oral surgery and applies mercury and nickel amalgams. In addition to these jobs, she cleans work surfaces using wipes containing quaternary ammonium compounds, and sterilizes dental equipment that she soaks in a proteinase subtilisin solution before sorting them into packets that are autoclaved in a heat sterilizer.

Her evaluation is significant for a methacholine challenge consistent with mild asthma, and routine prick skin tests negative to trees, grasses, weeds, cockroach, cat, dog, and molds, and positive to dust mites. Peak expiratory flow rate (PEFR) monitoring shows lower peak flows at work that improve on weekends and holidays. Repeat of a methacholine challenge at the end of a holiday period shows significantly less hyperresponsiveness than during a working period. Findings support a diagnosis of sensitizer-induced OA related to her current job.

As this case shows, however, exposures in any job can be complex, and may include any number of potential sensitizers that must be sorted through to identify the correct causative agent. Identification of the triggering exposures is based on patient history and the medical literature, and occasionally requires specialized testing. In this case, the presence of hives and asthma suggests that the patient's disease is allergic in nature, and likely caused by exposure to a high-molecular-weight (HMW) allergen at work. The patient reported that her hives were often specifically triggered by splashes from the enzyme solution when she placed dirty instruments into the plastic tub. She did not report skin or chest symptoms when working with dental impressions or dental alloys. Because her exposure was thought likely to be IgE-mediated and specifically related to a certain task, skin prick testing with the enzyme solution was performed and found to be positive.

HMW OA is asthma caused by sensitization to HMW, typically biologic, agents that produce disease through IgE-mediated mechanisms. Once the diagnosis of asthma is established and the work-relatedness of asthma has been determined, the pharmaceutical treatment of HMW-induced OA is the same as for non-OA and follows guidelines such as those by the NHLBI, last updated in 2007,[1] or GINA,[2] updated in 2009 (www.ginasthma.org). The next step is the identification and management of the causative exposure. Robust literature documents that the best medical outcomes for OA are produced by removal from exposure,[4–6] and in some patients asthma may then resolve. Predictors of improvement or resolution of asthma include fewer symptomatic years at work and better lung function at the time of diagnosis.[7,8] In many patients, however, asthma symptoms and need for treatment may persist long after the worker has left the workplace,[9,10] and specific reactivity to the immunologic agent persists even when nonspecific bronchial hyperresponsiveness has resolved.[11]

However, for many workers, removal from the job also brings significant social and economic costs.[12] An excellent summary of the socioeconomic impact of OA indicates that 25% to 38% of workers with immunologic OA have lost their jobs or been out of work for prolonged periods, and 42% to 78% report a substantial loss of income.[13] One study showed that factors keeping workers in their jobs include higher education level and income, age older than 40 years, longer years with the current employer, children to support, and exposure to an HMW agent (vs a low-molecular-weight [LMW] agent).[14] Asthma severity did not predict moving out of exposure or job in this review, although others have suggested this.[15]

The medical literature is inconsistent regarding the long-term outcomes of continued but reduced exposure to HMW allergens in workers with HMW OA compared with LMW OA, in which continued exposure usually leads to worsened disease. One small study following 10 workers with OA who were treated for asthma and remained in exposure showed no significant differences in lung function, use of rescue bronchodilator, or respiratory symptom scores over 3 years.[16] Two separate studies found similarly good outcomes in workers sensitized to natural rubber latex who were removed from exposure and those who remained in their jobs but greatly reduced their latex exposure through switching to nonlatex gloves while coworkers changed to low-protein powder-free latex gloves.[17,18] These studies indicate that when exposure modification is feasible, these patients may be able to remain in jobs with reduced exposure and with close medical follow-up. Exposure reduction is pivotal to allowing these patients to remain at work, and may be achieved through a switch to less-exposed jobs, improved worksite ventilation, use of alternate materials, and/or use of respiratory protection.[19] In these cases, however, close medical monitoring is mandatory to remaining in reduced exposure, so that the worker can be removed from exposure expeditiously if symptoms or lung function deteriorate. Patients should clearly understand that the chance of their asthma clearing or significantly improving diminishes as they remain exposed to the relevant sensitizer for long periods.

In this case, the patient decided to remain in her job, despite a long discussion as to possible health risks. The approach then was to treat her asthma, restrict her from direct or indirect exposure to the enzyme bath, and follow her clinically. The enzyme bath, located in a separate "dirty" room, was covered with a plastic lid, and the patient's job duties were modified so that she was no longer required to place dirty instruments in the bath to soak or remove them to package for autoclaving. She was started on treatment with a high-dose inhaled steroid, a rescue inhaler, and an antihistamine. She continued to follow her PEFRs at work and at home, and these improved to her normal baseline, with no significant excursions at work or at home. Exposure to other allergens and irritants in her workplace did not trigger decrements in her peak flows, indicating that these exposures did not have to be managed. Her hives resolved out of exposure. The patient was initially seen on a monthly basis for 6 months, which was then extended to every 2 to 3 months once she was found to be clinically stable.

For a few causes of HMW asthma, immunotherapy, when given in the context of medical monitoring, is a potential management choice. The ability to use immunotherapy to treat OA is very limited by few commercially available and relevant extracts, and very few studies showing efficacy. Some benefit has been seen with immunotherapy to latex in sensitized health care workers,[20] but this is not practical in the United States, where a latex extract has not yet been approved by the U.S. Food and Drug Administration, and usually is not required because removal of powdered latex gloves resolves disease.[21–23] Immunotherapy with hymenoptera venom in beekeepers and outdoor workers is clearly indicated when this diagnosis is confirmed; for other allergens, such as wheat flour in bakers, cat allergen in veterinarians, and laboratory animal allergens in researchers and animal handlers, evidence is based on only small, nonrandomized studies.[3,24,25]

Thus, for patients who elect to remain in their jobs with restricted or reduced exposure to the HMW occupational allergens found to cause their asthma, close medical surveillance is essential. If the patient's asthma remains stable or, preferably, improves on adequate medical management and restriction from exposure, then remaining in their job would seem to be safe. However, if treatment and exposure restrictions are not adequate to control the patient's asthma, then close medical surveillance will reveal the need to further restrict or remove the patient from the job. Requisites for remaining in the job include settings where the asthma is not severe, exposures can be effectively controlled, where patients can be closely followed, and agree that they will leave the job if their physician recommends removal because of worsening asthma. Not all workers with HMW OA can continue to perform the same job with removal from exposure to the causative allergen. This exposure may be an essential component of their jobs, or indirect exposures may remain high enough to trigger decrements in lung function and increases in medication needs despite no direct work with the causative agent. These workers may then need to obtain different work (preferably supported by workers' compensation for any associated income loss and costs for retraining).

One aspect of OA management that may be daunting for the allergy practitioner is how to initiate the dialog with the patient's workplace about restricting exposures. Communication between the physician and the workplace can only be initiated with the patient's written consent unless the patient has been referred by their workplace or through an occupational medicine physician under their worker's compensation insurance. In that case, the treating physician is able to provide information to the referral source regarding restrictions from certain exposures or specific jobs at work. Practitioners must be specific, because providing restrictions that are too broad may result in patients being unable to perform the essential functions of their job, and in the case of specific sensitization, only one or a few exposures need to be managed.

Furthermore, a new case of OA to an HMW or LMW sensitizer (the sentinel case) often indicates that coworkers may also be exposed and may be affected. If patients provide appropriate authorization, then treating physicians may be able to contact the health and safety organization responsible for managing these issues at the company, or a government agency, such as Occupational Safety and Health Administration (OSHA) in the United States or a provincial Ministry of Labour in Canada. Physicians who are seriously concerned about work conditions at a specific job site may contact the government agency without identifying the patient.

Prevention of sensitizer-induced OA

Primary prevention of HMW and LMW asthma requires identification of potential workplace sensitizers, and is based on restricting exposures to levels below which sensitization does not occur, or substituting agents that are not sensitizers. If these steps are not technologically possible, then secondary prevention involves medical monitoring of exposed workers for early detection of disease and removal from exposure. A recent report of a model of intervention strategies to reduce the incidence of OA and allergy in bakers found that the best outcomes were achieved through rigorous exposure reductions and a robust health surveillance program that identified sensitized workers early and reduced their individual exposures by 90%. Preemployment screening, in contrast, was not effective.[26]

Medical follow-back

In the United States, follow-back (ie, moving from the specific case to addressing exposure identification and control, and medical surveillance of other exposed workers) is often problematic, because it involves the intersection of private industry and government regulatory agencies. Effective surveillance for occupational disease requires follow-up activities to address exposures causing the disease. The intervention model, the Sentinel Event Notification System for Occupational Risk (SENSOR), joins occupational disease surveillance with state OSHA programs and enforcement inspections. Under this program, reporting a sentinel case of OA is sufficient to trigger OSHA intervention, and worker agreement for the inspections is not required, because the worker's identity is kept confidential. Not all states have access to this type of program, which nonetheless provides a potential model for effective intervention and follow-back.[27,28] This model is schematized in **Fig. 1**.

LMW SENSITIZER-INDUCED ASTHMA
Case Example

A 54-year-old man with no history of asthma or seasonal allergies has worked for 14 years as a machine operator for a company making quality engineered metal clamping and fastening systems for pipelines, light fixtures, auto tire pressure sensors, and the space shuttle. The process involves cutting parts out of coils of stainless steel, nickel copper, or nickel chromium alloy by machine. Parts are then further shaped and machined, sprayed with a coating powder, glued together, or printed with ink. The patient's chest symptoms began approximately 10 years earlier with the onset of chest tightness, wheezing in cold air, and nocturnal awakening with shortness of breath. At the time, he was working on a machine that made stainless steel ties for automobiles. His symptoms occurred at work and resolved on weekends or away

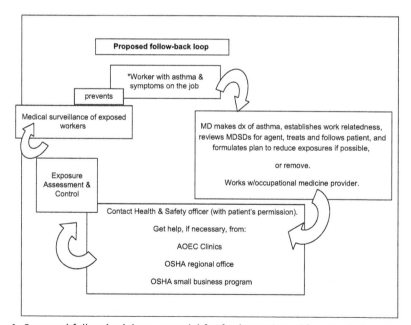

Fig. 1. Proposed follow-back loop: a model for further action with suspected work-related asthma.

on vacation. In 2006 he was admitted for treatment to the intensive care unit for a severe respiratory exacerbation, and he was diagnosed with asthma. Treatment with prednisone and inhaled steroids improved but did not resolve his symptoms. The patient's skin rash began approximately 2 years before evaluation, and was characterized as tiny, intensely itchy bumps located on hands, arms, and upper chest that blistered with yellow drainage over a week's time before resolving, and usually improved with topical steroids. Although the patient was moved to work on different machines, these were clustered together so that workers were indirectly exposed to a variety of different work processes and products in addition to their own job duties, and individual exposures could not be effectively reduced. Because the patient's asthma and skin rash were worsening despite adequate medical treatment, he was sent for further evaluation to determine a potential work-related cause. A methacholine challenge was positive for severe airway hyperresponsiveness. Skin prick testing was negative to all environmental allergens tested.

LMW sensitizers are typically defined as smaller molecules that can cause skin or respiratory diseases similarly to HMW antigens, but often through non-IgE based mechanisms. Most are highly reactive molecules that may become neoantigens after conjugating to epithelial proteins or to serum proteins such as albumin. After establishing the diagnosis of asthma, confirming the work-relatedness, and beginning asthma therapy, the correct management of LMW OA begins with the accurate identification of the causative agents. This scenario, based on a real case, shows that most workers have a complex set of exposures that can include several sensitizers. In many cases of LMW OA, diagnostic tools to determine sensitization, such as skin prick testing, in vitro–specific IgE testing, or patch testing, are not available to identify the specific sensitizing agent. A careful history, together with knowledge of the medical literature, is important for identifying relevant exposures for further testing. In this case, the patient identified several single component glues that seemed to trigger his rash and shortness of breath at work. The rash was most consistent with a contact dermatitis, and patch testing to glues used by the patient in the workplace elicited delayed responses to a polyglycol dimethacrylate and a second glue containing methyl 2-cyanoacrylate. Both compounds have been reported to cause contact dermatitis and OA.[29,30]

Peak flow monitoring showed normal PEFRs on weekends, and occasional but dramatic declines in peak flows from 480 L/min in the morning to 300 L/min in the evening by the end of the work week. Several times a week, the patient reported awakening from sleep with a PEFR of 240 L/min.

The patient was reluctant to leave his job, where he had been working for 14 years, because he earned a good salary without a high school diploma. However, the layout of the work processes was such that all work was performed in a large open warehouse on machines that were grouped together, and where specific exposures could not be reduced or modified. The patient asked whether he could remain in his job while using a respirator. Use of respirators requires specific fit testing, the availability of the right respirator to exclude the specific exposures of concern, and the physical capability of wearing the respirator during job exposures. In this case, given the widespread use of glues by many coworkers, the patient would have to wear a respirator for his entire work shift, which is generally not feasible. Cartridge-based respirators are often hot and uncomfortable, and impede communication with coworkers. In the case of allergen-driven asthma, a dust mask could not sufficiently exclude allergic exposures to protect him. Glue or other sensitizers could also adhere to his work clothes, providing another route of exposure. A powered air-purifying respirator is more comfortable but is expensive and not always protective in jobs requiring much physical movement. Respiratory protection is only reasonable in work settings that require the respirator to be worn for only limited periods, for an exposure that can be managed with a respirator, and when dermal exposure is not a concern. This option was not practicable for this patient, who ultimately required removal from the workplace. The decision was based on the impressive changes of the patient's PEFR at work, the severity of his symptoms, extent of his bronchial hyperresponsiveness, and the inability to effectively modify or reduce exposures. The severity of the patient's asthma, on treatment would make, leaving him in the workplace a medically risky decision.

The published medical literature documents a few examples of patients sensitized to LMW antigens who remained in their jobs with medical follow-up. One study of 25 patients with OA, of whom 22 had asthma caused by an LMW chemical, showed no significant differences in the percentage of predicted forced expiratory volume in 1 second or methacholine PD20 compared with baseline for the 12 patients who remained in their jobs, or the 13 with more severe disease who left employment.[15] Nonetheless, the outcome of LMW asthma in patients who are not removed from exposure is often one involving persistent symptoms, need for medication, and bronchial hyperresponsiveness, as in isocyanate-induced asthma[31,32] and western red cedar asthma.[4,33] A review of 10 fatal asthma cases identified isocyanates, a common LMW antigen, as the cause in 3.[34] In contrast, most workers with trimellitic anhydride (TMA) asthma who moved to jobs with lower exposures had improved symptoms, improved pulmonary functions, and lower IgE against TMA conjugated with human serum albumin. Those who did not improve with transfer to low-exposure jobs improved after transfer to jobs with no TMA exposure.[35]

Not all sensitizer-induced OA improves out of exposure.[3] Therefore, the patient should continue to be monitored for asthma symptom control, adequate dose of medications, and improvement in lung function after removal from exposure. The issue of other exposed workers and the management of workplace exposures should be addressed in a similar way as for HMW-induced OA.

IRRITANT-INDUCED OA
Case Example

A 40-year-old man who had never smoked and had no background history of asthma, respiratory disease, or allergic symptoms had worked for 10 years at a company that manufactured plastics. When the machinery was purged for cleaning, production was stopped and the area was evacuated to avoid exposure of workers to the irritating fumes. On one occasion when this was being undertaken, the worker had not been informed and walked into the area after his lunch break. He immediately noted strong fumes and a burning sensation in his eyes, nose, and throat with coughing. He left the area within a few minutes but developed progressive shortness of breath, wheeze, and cough. He was taken from work to the emergency department and was found to have tachypnea, wheezing on chest auscultation, and mild hypoxemia (oxygen saturation on room air, 89%). He was treated in the emergency department with supplemental oxygen, bronchodilators, and oral corticosteroids with good response and was discharged on inhaled corticosteroids and bronchodilators. He was initially out of work because of his symptoms for 3 weeks and then returned to his usual work with medical monitoring of his symptoms, medication needs, and serial peak flow readings. Pulmonary function tests and methacholine challenge 2 weeks after the exposure showed typical findings of asthma.

He continued to have asthma symptoms for the next 10 months, and found that he needed to use extra bronchodilator at work only during times of increased physical exertion or if the levels of dust and fumes were higher than usual. The methacholine PC20, which had been 0.4 mg/mL at first testing, progressively improved to 12 mg/mL 1 year later when symptoms had cleared. His asthma medications were adjusted with his improvement according to guidelines and he was able to stop medications at the end of the year. He was advised that he may have a recurrence of asthma symptoms at times of upper respiratory infections and should then restart as-needed bronchodilators and regular inhaled steroids for periods up to 6 weeks for significant symptoms at that time. Safety measures at work were reviewed to ensure that this worker and others would not have a similar accidental exposure to the acids. A claim was submitted to the workers' compensation system for reactive airway dysfunction syndrome (RADS) and was accepted. He received compensation for 3 weeks of lost time and the cost of his asthma medications, and was deemed to have minimal permanent impairment as a result of the exposure.

Management of RADS and irritant-induced OA

After the diagnosis of RADS or irritant-induced asthma, management aspects include pharmacologic treatment, exposure issues, and compensation, and consideration of other workers.[3,36] The pharmacologic management of RADS and less-definitive forms of irritant-induced asthma has generally followed asthma guidelines.[1,2] Because this condition results from irritant inflammatory responses, practitioners have assumed that corticosteroid use might be of benefit, and generally early treatment with corticosteroids is advised. Because of the accidental and sporadic nature of the exposures, usually affecting small numbers of workers at a time, controlled trials have not been performed to objectively evaluate any additional benefit of systemic corticosteroids compared with inhaled corticosteroids. Commonly, however, oral corticosteroids are given to patients with RADS or irritant-induced asthma, especially when they present acutely to the emergency department or an urgent care facility, in addition to inhaled steroids, bronchodilators, and general supportive measures as appropriate. A few case reports suggest more rapid improvement may occur with oral corticosteroid use.[37,38] Results of small case series have suggested[39] that patients with RADS show less bronchodilator responsiveness compared with other cases of OA. No evidence is available to determine the effects of other medications, but one study suggested benefit from early use of inhaled bicarbonate after accidental exposure to chlorine.[40]

The time course of improvement is variable, and pharmacologic management should be adjusted according to symptomatic and physiologic responses. The criteria for RADS include continuing manifestations of asthma for at least 12 weeks, whereas for the broader definition of irritant-induced asthma, manifestations may clear in a shorter time.

Appropriate management of further work exposure can vary depending on the chance of another event occurring similar to the one that triggered RADS/irritant-induced asthma, the severity and course of the resulting asthma, the presence of ongoing respiratory triggers in the workplace, and the ability to control asthma with pharmacologic measures. At one extreme, if the initial triggering event is not likely to recur, if the resulting asthma is mild and well controlled with inhaled medications, and if the work environment does not include triggers that may be expected to exacerbate asthma (eg, temperature extremes, humidity, strenuous exertion, dusts, smoke, fumes), then the patient may be able to return to the workplace without difficulty. However, if the resulting asthma is not well controlled with appropriate asthma medications and the work environment includes potential asthma triggers, then the patient may require initial time off from work for stabilization of asthma and to assess extent of improvement, and then may have a graduated return to work with medical monitoring of symptoms, medication needs, and peak flows and/or spirometry. The patient should initially start work in an area with the least exposure to expected asthma triggers and, for any short-term potential irritant exposures, use a suitable fit-tested respiratory protective device. If this work is well tolerated and there is a need to move back to an area with greater potential exposure, then this may be similarly assessed with medical monitoring. Over time, if asthma improves and airway responsiveness lessens, the patient may be able to return to usual work.

Workers' compensation programs in Canada and in the United States would generally provide support for work-induced RADS/irritant-induced asthma to assist in income replacement, medication costs, and, for persisting disease, long-term disability awards. Comorbidities can occur from the same accident that causes RADS/irritant-induced asthma, as was seen among workers at the site of the World Trade Center collapse, where the comorbidities included posttraumatic stress disorder; upper airway irritant syndromes, such as rhinitis and vocal cord dysfunction[41,42]; and additional lower airway disease besides asthma, such as bronchitis, bronchiolitis, and bronchiectasis.[43,44] Symptoms resulting from these and other syndromes, such as work-related irritable larynx syndrome,[45] may mimic asthma and should be carefully investigated to allow accurate diagnosis and treatment. Failure to identify these may lead to inappropriate overtreatment of apparently "unmanageable asthma."

Prognosis is highly variable. Asthma may persist for years, or symptoms may clear within months. A systematic review[46] reported a mean duration of 13 months (interquartile range, 6.5–43.5 months), but a report from a specialized OA center[47] described patients who had been followed up for a mean of almost 14 years: all had ongoing symptoms, most (68%) requiring inhaled corticosteroids, and only 6 of 23 had normalized their methacholine response. Predictive prognostic factors have not been identified.

Primary prevention of RADS/irritant-induced asthma requires a focus on best safety practices in the workplace for accident prevention. Training and ready availability of fit-tested appropriate respiratory protective devices for use in situations of high irritant exposures, and good occupational hygiene measures at work[3] will also help prevent disease. After an accidental spill or other high exposure, the conditions that led to the accident should be reviewed, and measures put in place to minimize further similar occurrence. Tertiary prevention to minimize disability comprises careful assessment and management of the affected workers.

WEA

Case Example with Very Transient WEA

A 37-year-old hospital cleaner had a history of perennial asthma and allergic rhinitis since childhood, which was worse during the summer and fall months, on exposure to animals, and at times of colds. Previous allergy skin tests had been positive to grass and ragweed pollens, dust mites, and animal extracts. She had no animals at home, used air conditioning during the summer, and generally had good control of her asthma with low-dose regular inhaled steroids and occasional use of her short-acting bronchodilator. She usually had no difficulty performing her usual work as a cleaner in the outpatient clinic area.

For 1 week during the vacation of a coworker, she was asked by her supervisor to transfer her work area and clean the medical ward, where stronger cleaning products, including bleach, were needed to clean patient mattresses and floors. Within two shifts of starting this work, she had to leave because of an exacerbation of her asthma that began after 20 minutes of using these cleaning products. Her asthma worsened the next day with further exposure, and did not respond to her regular medications. She then went to a walk-in clinic, where she was given a 2-day course of prednisone, although no pulmonary function testing was performed. She was out of work for the next 2 days before returning to her usual work area with no further problems. She elected not to submit a claim to the workers' compensation system for the 2 days of lost work because these were covered by her sickness insurance.

WEA Case Example with Frequent Work-Related Symptoms

A 19-year-old man had a history of asthma and eczema since infancy and had required several emergency visits and hospital admissions during childhood for his asthma, mainly at times of apparent viral upper respiratory tract infections. He also had symptoms of allergic rhinitis and exacerbation of asthma on exposure to cats and dust, and had positive skin prick tests to cats and dust mites. During his teenage years, his asthma was well controlled with avoidance of cats, dust mite control measures, and use of a regular combined steroid and long-acting bronchodilator. He then seldom needed to use his short-acting bronchodilator except at times of colds.

He began work in a foundry but almost immediately noted worsening of his asthma symptoms, and needed to use his short-acting bronchodilator several times during each working day. He noted improvement during weekends and holidays. His work required him to carry heavy loads in a hot humid environment, with exposure to fumes and dusts (but no identified respiratory sensitizers). He was unable to tolerate use of a respiratory protective device because of the heat and humidity in the workplace. Despite an increase in his inhaled steroid dosage and a trial of a leukotriene inhibitor, his asthma remained poorly controlled in this job and he frequently had to leave work early because of his symptoms. Evaluation with serial peak flow readings and symptom/medication monitoring during periods of working and holidays confirmed his history of worsening asthma at work. Spirometry at the end of a work week showed more severe airflow limitation compared with the end of a holiday period, but methacholine challenge and induced sputum eosinophil results did not differ significantly at the end of his holiday and the end of a working week.

He was diagnosed with WEA and was advised that he should work in a cleaner environment with moderate temperature and humidity, and limited exposure to dusts, fumes, and sprays. He received support from his local workers' compensation system for WEA, and obtained a job in a convenience store. After leaving the foundry his asthma symptoms were again well controlled with use of a regular combined steroid and long-acting bronchodilator and, as before the foundry job, he seldom needed to use his short-acting bronchodilator except at times of colds. He did, however, experience a reduction in hourly wage in his new job compared with his work in the foundry, and had to move from his rented apartment back to live with his parents until he could find a better-paying job.

Management of WEA

As illustrated with these two cases, WEA can range from a single transient episode at work that may lead to very little or no income loss or lost time from work, to very significant morbidity resulting in loss of time from work and reduction in income. Most population-based or primary care surveys, and a review of cases from a workers' compensation system that accepted claims for WEA, suggest that transient symptoms of WEA are the most common.[48–51] In contrast, tertiary care clinic population studies have mostly included patients with more frequent or persisting symptoms, as may be expected.[52–54]

The management will vary depending on the individual circumstances. For patients with a transient single exacerbation of asthma at work, performing objective tests to document the episode is usually not feasible. Commonly these patients are not seen by a specialist at the time of the exacerbation, but may visit a primary health care provider or an emergency department for acute asthma management, where they are treated according to the severity of the asthma exacerbation as recommended by asthma guidelines. Ideally, pulmonary function testing would be performed at that visit. In the absence of pulmonary function tests from the time of the exacerbation to compare with results from before or after the asthma flare, a presumptive diagnosis of WEA is generally reached from the history of an exposure at work that may be expected to exacerbate asthma, worsened asthma symptoms in a patient with a previous diagnosis of asthma, and increased need for asthma medication at that time.

Conversely, if worsened asthma symptoms occur frequently at work, then objective documentation should be obtained. As suggested in the recent American College of Chest Physicians consensus document,[3] triggering exposures at work should be identified, the diagnosis of asthma should be confirmed objectively, and the work relationship established by serial symptom records, medication needs, and peak expiratory flow rates during periods at and away from work. When feasible, spirometry, methacholine challenges, and induced sputum cytology assessed near the end of a working period should be compared with results at the end of a period off work to provide a better understanding of the relationship to work exposures. Immunologic tests to document the presence of specific IgE antibodies to work sensitizers and to common environmental allergens may also clarify the diagnosis. A full clinical evaluation of asthma is important, particularly in patients who have frequent or more severe exacerbations.

A combination of external contributing factors may be present in addition to the work exposure, and understanding these can facilitate management. For example, a stone cutter who works outdoors and is allergic to grass pollen notes significant exacerbations of asthma only when he is exposed to fine dust from cutting stone in May and June each year. He has no difficulty with this work at other times of the year, and no difficulty on weekends outdoors in May and June when he is not cutting stone. Therefore, a full history, including occupational and nonoccupational exposures and triggers to asthma, medication use and adherence, and allergy skin testing, should be obtained. Additional diagnoses that may coexist and exacerbate or mimic asthma symptoms, such as work-related irritable larynx syndromes,[45] other upper airway syndromes, seasonal allergies, and gastroesophageal reflux disease, should also be treated. When these nonoccupational factors affecting asthma can be identified and managed, then workplace triggers may contribute less to asthma worsening.

If the presumed triggering exposure was an unusual event at work that is not likely to recur, then the patient may resume their usual work while taking optimal asthma medications. Similarly, if the exposure is common but the asthma exacerbation only occurred when the patient had underlying poor control of asthma (eg, had run out of inhaled steroid medication, had a concurrent upper respiratory infection), then asthma education and optimized medical management (including an increase of medication in association with presumed viral upper respiratory infections) should improve asthma control so that a change in work exposures may not be needed.

However, if an exacerbating exposure is likely to be recurrent (eg, the use of stronger cleaning agents in a patient care area for the first WEA case example, or dusts and fumes in the foundry for the second WEA case example) and symptoms have occurred or are likely to occur more frequently, then further action is likely needed. In cases when a likely asthma trigger could easily be avoided, an option is to provide the patient with a note to give to the employer advising future avoidance of that trigger (an accommodation that would not be difficult for the employer of the first WEA case). This solution also may be practical for patients with asthma transiently exacerbated during one-time exposures at work, such as office renovations or during occasional events such as office floor wax stripping or waxing. However, providing accommodations to avoid exposure would be very difficult in other settings (as for the second WEA case), and significant work changes may be necessary. An approach to determining whether the patient can continue at work would be to first optimize pharmacologic medical treatment for asthma, then medically monitor the patient in the workplace. Monitoring should include self-reported diaries of symptoms, medication needs, and serial peak flow recordings obtained before and during a trial of exposure reduction using occupational hygiene measures and appropriate personal protective equipment. The addition of spirometry, methacholine challenges, and, where available, induced sputum cytology before and at the end of this trial can further provide objective assessment of the effects of job modifications on the patient's asthma.

An additional differential diagnosis that may affect management is that of OA in patients who have no history of asthma before starting the job. In these instances, whether asthma started coincidentally while working and is exacerbated by work factors or if it is caused by work (OA) is unclear. Many workplaces include exposures to both potential sensitizers and nonspecific irritant agents capable of causing or exacerbating asthma. Immunologic tests showing specific IgE antibodies to a work sensitizer are more supportive of OA. However, other tests, such as serial symptoms, medications and peak flow recordings, demonstration of worsening airway responsiveness to methacholine, or increased sputum eosinophilia during a work period compared with an off-work period, may not distinguish OA from WEA.[52,55] Specific laboratory challenges with the suspected sensitizer may be needed for a more definitive diagnosis. If specific sensitization to a work agent is identified, then the management is as described for sensitizer-induced OA.

Specific sensitization to an agent specific to the workplace can also occur in patients with preexisting asthma. When this is identified, the management of the patient is the same as for sensitizer-induced OA (although no general consensus exists as to whether this condition should be classified as OA or WEA).

Finally, common environmental aeroallergens can also be present at work and exacerbate asthma, such as pollen and seasonal fungal spores for outdoor workers, and dust mites and cat allergens for domestic cleaners. When these exposures worsen asthma in patients with underlying or preexisting asthma, then this is usually regarded as WEA.[3] However, avoidance of specific allergens may need to be more stringent than the reduction of exposure that is adequate for less-specific triggers, such as fumes, sprays, and temperature extremes. In addition, the effects of an allergic asthmatic response can be associated with late-phase inflammatory responses and more prolonged increases in airway hyperresponsiveness than are generally associated with nonimmune, trigger exposures. Therefore these responses must be identified and managed with greater levels of avoidance and careful monitoring to ensure a safe work environment. Allergen immunotherapy is also a consideration for responses to common aeroallergens.

Although it is important to ensure that workplace exposures are within the allowable occupational limits, exposure monitoring currently has little benefit in the management of WEA. An exposure can be well within allowable safe levels for most workers who do not have asthma, but can still be at an exacerbating level for those with airway hyperresponsiveness.[3] Similarly, an immunologic response in the airways can occur with exposures even below the monitoring detection limit. Nevertheless, occupational hygiene measures should be optimized so that the entire workforce exposures to irritant respiratory agents are limited as much as possible.[3] Respiratory protective devices are not comfortable to wear for prolonged periods, and for those with underlying rhinitis and asthma, they may not be well tolerated, and compliance may be poor.[56] In general, respiratory protective devices are only recommended for short-term use when exposure levels are increased.

Workers' compensation is available in some (but not all) areas to provide some support to those with WEA (personal communication, 2011). Despite attempts to modify and reduce exposure to exacerbating triggers, some patients may not be able to continue to work with the same employer without ongoing exacerbation of their asthma. If they are not supported by a workers' compensation system, they may need short-term or long-term disability support. Outcome assessments have suggested poor socioeconomic outcomes for those seen in a tertiary referral center with WEA, similar to those with OA.

Preventive measures for WEA include both workplace and patient measures. Workplace prevention includes minimizing respiratory irritant exposures in work settings, safety training, and appropriate use of fit-tested and readily available respiratory protective devices when needed. Patient directed preventive measures include (1) optimal asthma management strategies, including control of exposure to nonoccupational triggers, education, and medication use, (2) recognition of, and education on, the potential for WEA, and (3) appropriate actions to take. Education of young asthmatics before starting work may increase awareness and understanding of asthma triggers in the general environment and in work settings, and ways to control exposures. Recent studies suggest that young asthmatics seldom discuss their career plans with their physicians,[57] and most do not consider their asthma when making career choices.[57,58] In addition to their risk of WEA from nonspecific asthma triggers at work, those with underlying atopy have been shown to have an increased risk of developing sensitization at work to allergens such as laboratory animal allergens, natural rubber latex, and bakery allergens. Although they should not be excluded from these occupations, their increased risk may justify more intensive educational efforts[59] and possibly more intensive medical surveillance measures if they choose these occupations.

Overview of Workers' Compensation Systems

In the United States, workers' compensation systems are state-based, and therefore differ somewhat among states. In most states, employers must buy workers' compensation insurance to treat work-related injuries and illnesses in their employees. If workers have sustained an injury or illness, such as asthma, which they attribute to the workplace, they must notify their employer and file a first report of injury through their employer. That report is then filed with the workers' compensation insurance carrier, which assigns a case number and a date of injury. The worker is then typically seen by occupational medicine physicians contracted by the employer, although in several states employees may see their personal physician. In most states, the first physician to see the patient must file a standard report form with the insurer, which includes the diagnosis, treatment plan, work-relatedness, and work restrictions. At each visit, the patient's physical status is assessed, treatment is documented, the physician provides restrictions to job duties or exposures that might aggravate the injury or illness, and schedules a return visit to assess progress. If patients are restricted from their job or the workplace by their physician, then they may receive temporary total disability (TTD) pay during that time, typically two-thirds of their usual wage. If the employer contests the claim, stating that the injury or illness is not work-related, then the worker does not receive TTD and the situation becomes contentious.

In many cases, states provide treatment guidelines for different kinds of injuries, although guidelines for occupational respiratory diseases are not yet available. If the occupational medicine physician determines that information from a specialist is needed, then approval is obtained from the workers' compensation carrier to refer the patient for further testing and treatment. The referral physician also needs to obtain the workers' compensation carrier's approval for any further testing necessary to establish the diagnosis or assess treatment response.

Two aspects of this process differ from conventional medicine. The primary goal is to treat patients until they can return to their job, and patients are typically seen very frequently, such as once a week, to get them back to work. The second aspect is the emphasis on determining the causative exposure, such as whether it is ergonomic, inhalational, or dermal. If the exposure can be modified or removed, then the worker has a greater chance of successfully returning to work once the treating physician determines that the patient has reached maximum medical improvement (MMI), meaning the patient has received all management that can be reasonably expected to improve their condition. Concordance with treatment guidelines also helps determine when the patient is at MMI. In terms of OA caused by a sensitizer, the recommendation is for patients to remain 2 years out of exposure with adequate treatment before being considered at MMI. Once at MMI, the patient's medical treatment benefits are terminated and they no longer receive TTD pay.

At that point, the patient undergoes an impairment rating, which in many states is determined using specific guidelines provided by the American Medical Association in the AMA Guides to the Evaluation of Permanent Impairment, according to organ system. In general, impairment is based on interference with activities of daily living, need for ongoing treatment, and objective measures of limitation, which may include range of motion for musculoskeletal impairment, or response to bronchodilator or methacholine reactivity for OA. The AMA OA guidelines are largely based on the American Thoracic Society guidelines for the evaluation of impairment/disability in patients with asthma.[60] In a few states physicians are required to obtain accreditation through courses provided by their state Division of Workers' Compensation or other training entities to be certified to perform impairment ratings. Specialists can frequently provide guidance regarding adequate medical management, removal or modification of exposure, and need for ongoing treatment.

In Canada, each province has a separate workers' compensation system with slightly different claim mechanisms and support (Ontario is one of the few systems that accept claims for WEA and OA but usually provides a lesser extent of support for this). Details of claim submissions and support are available on the provincial system Web sites. A claim can be initiated by either the affected worker, the employer, or the physician. After one of these parties submits the initial form, the other two are required to submit additional information. The worker is asked to sign a release of information form to permit release of all relevant medical records to the compensation system. A claim decision may be reached based on the information received, or the compensation system may request an additional referral to a specialist for further investigations or expert opinion. Acceptance of a claim for OA can provide economic support for lost income, costs of required asthma medications, retraining in some cases for labor market reentry, and compensation for noneconomic loss (disability), usually assessed when maximum medical recovery is expected to have occurred.

SUMMARY

Management strategies for work-related asthma vary with the category of work-related asthma, and also, to some extent, differ depending on individual factors. In general, those with OA from a work sensitizer are advised to avoid further exposure to that agent when feasible, whereas those with OA caused by an irritant exposure and those with WEA (if not triggered by a specific allergen/sensitizer) can often continue to work in the same company but may require some reduction in exposure to workplace asthma triggers.

REFERENCES

1. National Asthma Education and Prevention Program. Expert Panel Report 3 (EPR-3): guidelines for the diagnosis and management of asthma-summary report 2007. J Allergy Clin Immunol 2007;120(Suppl 5):S94–138.
2. Bateman ED, Hurd SS, Barnes PJ, et al. Global strategy for asthma management and prevention: GINA executive summary. Eur Respir J 2008;31(1):143–78.
3. Tarlo SM, Balmes J, Balkissoon R, et al. Diagnosis and management of work-related asthma: American College Of Chest Physicians Consensus Statement. Chest 2008;134(Suppl 3):1S–41S.
4. Chan-Yeung M, MacLean L, Paggiaro PL. Follow-up study of 232 patients with occupational asthma caused by western red cedar (Thuja plicata). J Allergy Clin Immunol 1987;79(5):792–6.
5. Pisati G, Baruffini A, Zedda S. Toluene diisocyanate induced asthma: outcome according to persistence or cessation of exposure. Br J Ind Med 1993;50(1): 60–4.
6. Merget R, Schulte A, Gebler A, et al. Outcome of occupational asthma due to platinum salts after transferral to low-exposure areas. Int Arch Occup Environ Health 1999;72(1):33–9.
7. Tarlo SM, Banks D, Liss G, et al. Outcome determinants for isocyanate induced occupational asthma among compensation claimants. Occup Environ Med 1997;54(10):756–61.
8. Maghni K, Lemiere C, Ghezzo H, et al. Airway inflammation after cessation of exposure to agents causing occupational asthma. Am J Respir Crit Care Med 2004;169(3):367–72.
9. Allard C, Cartier A, Ghezzo H, et al. Occupational asthma due to various agents. Absence of clinical and functional improvement at an interval of four or more years after cessation of exposure. Chest 1989;96(5):1046–9.
10. Lemiere C, Cartier A, Dolovich J, et al. Outcome of specific bronchial responsiveness to occupational agents after removal from exposure. Am J Respir Crit Care Med 1996;154(2 Pt 1):329–33.
11. Lemiere C, Cartier A, Malo JL, et al. Persistent specific bronchial reactivity to occupational agents in workers with normal nonspecific bronchial reactivity. Am J Respir Crit Care Med 2000;162(3 Pt 1):976–80.
12. Gannon PF, Weir DC, Robertson AS, et al. Health, employment, and financial outcomes in workers with occupational asthma. Br J Ind Med 1993;50(6):491–6.
13. Vandenplas O, Toren K, Blanc PD. Health and socioeconomic impact of work-related asthma. Eur Respir J 2003;22(4):689–97.
14. Miedinger D, Malo JL, Ghezzo H, et al. Factors influencing duration of exposure with symptoms and costs of occupational asthma. Eur Respir J 2010;36(4): 728–34.

15. Moscato G, Dellabianca A, Perfetti L, et al. Occupational asthma: a longitudinal study on the clinical and socioeconomic outcome after diagnosis. Chest 1999; 115(1):249–56.
16. Marabini A, Siracusa A, Stopponi R, et al. Outcome of occupational asthma in patients with continuous exposure: a 3-year longitudinal study during pharmacologic treatment. Chest 2003;124(6):2372–6.
17. Larbanois A, Jamart J, Delwiche JP, et al. Socioeconomic outcome of subjects experiencing asthma symptoms at work. Eur Respir J 2002;19(6):1107–13.
18. Bernstein DI, Biagini RE, Karnani R, et al. In vivo sensitization to purified Hevea brasiliensis proteins in health care workers sensitized to natural rubber latex. J Allergy Clin Immunol 2003;111(3):610–6.
19. Ameille J, Descatha A. Outcome of occupational asthma. Curr Opin Allergy Clin Immunol 2005;5(2):125–8.
20. Sastre J, Fernandez-Nieto M, Rico P, et al. Specific immunotherapy with a standardized latex extract in allergic workers: a double-blind, placebo-controlled study. J Allergy Clin Immunol 2003;111(5):985–94.
21. Tarlo SM, Easty A, Eubanks K, et al. Outcomes of a natural rubber latex control program in an Ontario teaching hospital. J Allergy Clin Immunol 2001;108(4): 628–33.
22. Charous BL, Blanco C, Tarlo S, et al. Natural rubber latex allergy after 12 years: recommendations and perspectives. J Allergy Clin Immunol 2002;109(1):31–4.
23. Allmers H, Schmengler J, Skudlik C. Primary prevention of natural rubber latex allergy in the German health care system through education and intervention. J Allergy Clin Immunol 2002;110(2):318–23.
24. Sastre J, Quirce S. Immunotherapy: an option in the management of occupational asthma? Curr Opin Allergy Clin Immunol 2006;6(2):96–100.
25. Quirce S, Sastre J. Recent advances in the management of occupational asthma. Expert Rev Clin Immunol 2008;4(6):757–65.
26. Meijster T, Warren N, Heederik D, et al. What is the best strategy to reduce the burden of occupational asthma and allergy in bakers? Occup Environ Med 2011;68(3):176–82.
27. Rosenman KD, Reilly MJ, Kalinowski DJ. A state-based surveillance system for work-related asthma. J Occup Environ Med 1997;39(5):415–25.
28. Reed PL, Rosenman K, Gardiner J, et al. Evaluating the Michigan SENSOR Surveillance Program for work-related asthma. Am J Ind Med 2007;50(9):646–56.
29. Moulin P, Magnan A, Lehucher-Michel MP. Occupational allergic contact dermatitis and asthma due to a single low molecular weight agent. J Occup Health 2009;51(1):91–6.
30. Sauni R, Kauppi P, Alanko K, et al. Occupational asthma caused by sculptured nails containing methacrylates. Am J Ind Med 2008;51(12):968–74.
31. Padoan M, Pozzato V, Simoni M, et al. Long-term follow-up of toluene diisocyanate-induced asthma. Eur Respir J 2003;21(4):637–40.
32. Piirila PL, Nordman H, Keskinen HM, et al. Long-term follow-up of hexamethylene diisocyanate-, diphenylmethane diisocyanate-, and toluene diisocyanate-induced asthma. Am J Respir Crit Care Med 2000;162(2 Pt 1):516–22.
33. Lin FJ, Dimich-Ward H, Chan-Yeung M. Longitudinal decline in lung function in patients with occupational asthma due to western red cedar. Occup Environ Med 1996;53(11):753–6.
34. Ortega HG, Kreiss K, Schill DP, et al. Fatal asthma from powdering shark cartilage and review of fatal occupational asthma literature. Am J Ind Med 2002; 42(1):50–4.

35. Grammer LC, Shaughnessy MA, Kenamore BD. Clinical and immunologic outcome of 42 individuals with trimellitic anhydride-induced immunologic lung disease after transfer to low exposure. Allergy Asthma Proc 2000;21(6):355–9.
36. Tarlo SM. Irritant-induced asthma. Pulmonary, and Critical Care and Sleep Update (PCCSU) 2010;24(Lesson 22).
37. Lemiere C, Malo JL, Boulet LP, et al. Reactive airways dysfunction syndrome induced by exposure to a mixture containing isocyanate: functional and histopathologic behaviour. Allergy 1996;51(4):262–5.
38. Lemiere C, Malo JL, Boutet M. Reactive airways dysfunction syndrome due to chlorine: sequential bronchial biopsies and functional assessment. Eur Respir J 1997;10(1):241–4.
39. Gautrin D, Boulet LP, Boutet M, et al. Is reactive airways dysfunction syndrome a variant of occupational asthma? J Allergy Clin Immunol 1994;93(1 Pt 1): 12–22.
40. Aslan S, Kandis H, Akgun M, et al. The effect of nebulized NaHCO3 treatment on "RADS" due to chlorine gas inhalation. Inhal Toxicol 2006;18(11):895–900.
41. Prezant DJ, Levin S, Kelly KJ, et al. Upper and lower respiratory diseases after occupational and environmental disasters. Mt Sinai J Med 2008;75(2):89–100.
42. Brackbill RM, Hadler JL, DiGrande L, et al. Asthma and posttraumatic stress symptoms 5 to 6 years following exposure to the World Trade Center terrorist attack. JAMA 2009;302(5):502–16.
43. Weiden MD, Ferrier N, Nolan A, et al. Obstructive airways disease with air trapping among firefighters exposed to World Trade Center dust. Chest 2010; 137(3):566–74.
44. de la Hoz RE. Long-term outcomes of acute irritant-induced asthma and World Trade Center-related lower airway disease. Am J Respir Crit Care Med 2010; 181(1):95–6.
45. Hoy RF, Ribeiro M, Anderson J, et al. Work-associated irritable larynx syndrome. Occup Med (Lond) 2010;60(7):546–51.
46. Shakeri MS, Dick FD, Ayres JG. Which agents cause reactive airways dysfunction syndrome (RADS)? A systematic review. Occup Med (Lond) 2008;58(3):205–11.
47. Malo JL, L'Archeveque J, Castellanos L, et al. Long-term outcomes of acute irritant-induced asthma. Am J Respir Crit Care Med 2009;179(10):923–8.
48. Buyantseva LV, Liss GM, Luce CE, et al. Work-aggravated asthma and occupational asthma in Ontario: relative frequency and exposures. Am J Respir Crit Care Med 2007;177:A804.
49. Henneberger PK. Work-exacerbated asthma. Curr Opin Allergy Clin Immunol 2007;7(2):146–51.
50. Henneberger PK, Derk SJ, Sama SR, et al. The frequency of workplace exacerbation among health maintenance organisation members with asthma. Occup Environ Med 2006;63(8):551–7.
51. Saarinen K, Karjalainen A, Martikainen R, et al. Prevalence of work-aggravated symptoms in clinically established asthma. Eur Respir J 2003;22(2):305–9.
52. Chiry S, Cartier A, Malo JL, et al. Comparison of peak expiratory flow variability between workers with work-exacerbated asthma and occupational asthma. Chest 2007;132(2):483–8.
53. Vandenplas O, Henneberger PK. Socioeconomic outcomes in work-exacerbated asthma. Curr Opin Allergy Clin Immunol 2007;7(3):236–41.
54. Santos MS, Jung H, Peyrovi J, et al. Occupational asthma and work-exacerbated asthma: factors associated with time to diagnostic steps. Chest 2007;131(6): 1768–75.

55. Girard F, Chaboillez S, Cartier A, et al. An effective strategy for diagnosing occupational asthma: use of induced sputum. Am J Respir Crit Care Med 2004;170(8): 845–50.
56. Rosenblat J, Fukakusa B, Jang B, et al. H1N1 fear rising for workers everywhere, but will they wear a mask? if not, why not? Chest 2009;136:47S.
57. Bhinder S, Cicutto L, Abdel-Qadir HM, et al. Perception of asthma as a factor in career choice among young adults with asthma. Can Respir J 2009;16(6): e69–75.
58. Radon K, Huemmer S, Dressel H, et al. Do respiratory symptoms predict job choices in teenagers? Eur Respir J 2006;27(4):774–8.
59. Radon K. To be or not to be: light at the end of the tunnel of career counseling for atopics. Am J Respir Crit Care Med 2008;177(8):806–7.
60. Guidelines for the evaluation of impairment/disability in patients with asthma. American Thoracic Society. Medical Section of the American Lung Association. Am Rev Respir Dis 1993;147(4):1056–61.

Irritant-Induced Airway Disorders

Stuart M. Brooks, MD[a],*, I. Leonard Bernstein, MD[b]

KEYWORDS

- Reactive airways dysfunction syndrome • RADS • Irritancy
- Ion channels • TRPV1 • TRPA1

Workplace exposures trigger or aggravate asthma principally by three links: (1) immunologic or allergic sensitization to a substance; (2) acute exposure to a high concentration of an irritant at work (nonallergic; reactive airways dysfunction syndrome [RADS]), or (3) exacerbation or aggravation of preexisting asthma.

Occupational asthma includes all types of asthma in the workplace, whether of immunologic or nonimmunologic origins. Work-related asthma, an analogous expression, is asthma exacerbated or induced by inhalational exposure in the workplace.[1] This term encompasses sensitizer-induced asthma and irritant-induced asthma.[2,3] Irritant-induced asthma is also referred to as occupational asthma without latency. Work-aggravated asthma corresponds to preexisting or concurrent asthma that is exacerbated or aggravated by workplace exposures to airborne irritant dusts, gases, vapors, or fumes.[4,5] Some clinicians differentiate between work-exacerbated asthma and work-aggravated asthma, based on whether the worker returns to a prior asthma baseline (ie, work-exacerbated asthma) or does not (work-aggravated asthma). However, this distinction is not accepted by everyone. Work-aggravated asthma may be the most common effect of work on asthma.[4] Up to 20% of full-time workers with asthma report work-aggravated asthma symptoms on a weekly basis.

Although thousands of people experience accidental high-level irritant exposures each year and seek medical care, most of them recover and few persons die.[6,7] Some individuals manifest residual impairment after an inhalation exposure that may take longer to resolve. Genetic reasons and host factors, such as cigarette smoking or preexisting lung diseases, purportedly come into play.[6,8,9]

Financial disclosures and/or conflicts of interest: The authors have nothing to disclose.

a Colleges of Public Health & Medicine, USF Health Science Center, University of South Florida, 13201 Bruce B. Downs Boulevard, Tampa, FL 33612, USA
b Division of Immunology, Allergy and Rheumatology, University of Cincinnati College of Medicine, 3255 Eden Avenue, Suite 350, ML 563, Cincinnati, OH 45267-0563, USA
* Corresponding author.
E-mail address: sbrooks@health.usf.edu

Immunol Allergy Clin N Am 31 (2011) 747–768
doi:10.1016/j.iac.2011.07.002
immunology.theclinics.com

IRRITANT, IRRITATION, AND ALLERGY

An irritant is a noncorrosive chemical that causes a reversible chemical inflammatory reaction on direct contact with the skin, eyes, nose, or respiratory system.[10,11] The actions of an irritant are nonspecific and do not entail an immunologic mechanism. Mechanistically, the effects may stem from an irritant's facility to react with different chemicals, such as sulfur or cysteine molecules, or form double bonds with human proteins.

Somesthesis, chemesthesis, and chemical nociception are terms to describe the chemically-stimulated feeling of an irritant.[12,13] Presumably, this chemosensory sensation plays some role as a warning system against exposure to irritant and potentially toxic exposures. The appreciation of irritation (ie, chemesthesis) affecting the eyes, nose, and throat is principally mediated by the trigeminal nerve (cranial nerve V). Pulmonary irritation is mainly controlled by the vagal (cranial nerve X) nerve.

Pungency refers to a sharp, bitter, or biting taste, but can also refer to an irritating odor.[14–16] Odor is detected by the olfactory nerve (cranial nerve I). The nose is not a sensitive discriminator for irritancy and odor does not equate with toxicity. There may be magnitudes of differences between the detection concentration of an airborne odorant and the concentration causing pungency, irritation, or even significant toxicity.[12,17]

Allergy occurs because there is an interaction with the immune system. It depends on the unique sensitivity of the person exposed to the allergen. Allergy is usually the result of prior repeated exposures to the allergen before there is the capacity for an immunologic or allergic response (ie, allergic sensitization). In contrast to an irritant, an allergen is often present in low concentrations.

Conversely, there may be a connection between an irritant exposure and allergy. Preexposure to an irritating air pollutant leads to greater airway responsiveness to an allergen to which the person is previously sensitized.[18] The human respiratory epithelium behaves as a physical barrier and a modulator of local airway inflammation.[19] Conceivably, the inflammation noted with irritancy occurs by the recruitment of Th_2 cytokine-producing cells, which amplify Th_2 inflammation through the induction of thymic stromal lymphopoietin.[20,21] Another example of an association between allergy and irritancy is when there is the deposition of an allergen enzyme on the surface of the respiratory mucosa; the process may incite local inflammation and enhance immunologic actions. Dust mite proteolytic allergens *Der p 1* and *Der p 9* trigger the release of IL-6, IL-8, and granulocyte-macrophage colony-stimulating factor from primary and secondary cultures of human bronchial epithelium in a dose-dependent and time-dependent manner.[19]

Stedman's Medical Dictionary refers to the state of irritation as being an "extreme incipient inflammatory reaction of the tissues to an injury."[21] Microscopically, a tissue's response to an irritant may show concentrations of inflammatory cells, vascular congestion, local increased blood flow, edema and plasma extravasation, and glandular hypersecretion. These pathologic tissue alterations translate clinically as redness and warmth, mucous hypersecretion, and local swelling. There is usually nervous hypersensitivity with, perhaps, a sensation of annoyance, discomfort, and/ or pain at the affected site. According to Shusterman,[22] the word irritation may have several meanings in the context of inhalation injury. The word may signify chemically induced respiratory tract damage; neurogenically mediated reflex changes in regional blood flow, mucus secretion, and airway caliber; or just a subjective sensation of airway irritation. Typically, the first lines of cells that come in contact with an irritant suffer the greatest injury.

There is no consensus as how to classify the pulmonary responses to irritants. Brooks[23] suggested classification according to the intensity of the irritant exposure (massive vs low or moderate), the differences in the physical properties of the irritant (halogenated vs nonhalogenated gas), the vapor pressure (when high, there are higher levels in air), solubility (determines upper vs lower airway distribution), the physical state (whether it is a vapor, gas fume, or dust), and chemical reactivity (highly reactive chemicals tend to be more irritating). Separating the irritant reaction according to the duration of the exposure is another approach. When the intensity of the irritant exposure is immense, the pulmonary outcome depends, in general, on whether there is proximal or distal pulmonary injury. **Table 1** reveals common causes of irritation in various situations and **Table 2** provides some consequences of irritant exposures.

IRRITANT-INDUCED ASTHMA

Irritant-induced asthma, also referred to as "asthma without latency,"[25] is a type of work-related asthma in which there is no recognized latency and no immunologic sensitization.[3,24–26] According to Lemière and colleagues,[27] the definition of irritant-induced asthma is limited to an asthmatic syndrome from single or multiple exposures to irritant products. When only a single exposure is responsible, the term RADS is used.

There are features that distinguish irritant-induced asthma from allergic occupational asthma.[28] Early on, coughing is a predominant symptom. Subsequently, bronchial obstruction, if present, does not respond well to bronchodilators.[28] The long-term outcome of subjects with irritant-induced asthma is at least as poor as that found in subjects with allergic occupational asthma.[28] There may be additional alteration from inhaling irritant gases and fumes. For example, obliterative bronchiolitis has been described in victims of the Bhopal accident.[29]

Table 1	
Common causes of irritation in various situations	
Exposure	**Agent or Process**
Acids	Glacial acetic, sulfuric, hydrochloric, hydrofluoric
Alkali	Bleach, calcium oxide, sodium hydroxide, World Trade Center dust, air bag emissions
Gases	Chlorine, sulfur dioxide, ammonia, mustard, ozone, hydrogen sulfide, phosgene, nitrogen dioxide
Sprays	Paints, coatings
Explosion	Irritant gases, vapors, fume releases under pressure
Fire or Pyrolysis	Combustion and pyrolysis products of fires, burning paint fumes, pyrolysis products of polyvinylchloride, meat-wrapping film
Confined Spaces	Epichlorohydrin, acrolein, floor sealant, metal-coating remover, biocides, fumigating aerosol, cleaning aerosol sprays, mixture of drain-cleaning agents
Workplace	Glass-bottle manufacture, popcorn flavoring manufacture, second-hand tobacco smoke, chlorine gas puffs, pyrite dust explosion, locomotive and diesel exhaust, aerosols of metalworking fluids, aluminum smelting (potroom fumes), metal processing, pulp milling, shoe and leather manufacture (organic solvents), exposure to SO2 from apricot sulfurization, aldehydes (formaldehyde, glutaraldehyde), biologic dusts, tunnel construction, coke oven emissions, food industry cleaners and disinfectants, chili pepper picking, cyanoacrylates

Table 2 Some consequences of irritant exposures	
Single, High-Level Exposure	**Repeated, Moderate-Level Exposure**
Upper airway edema and obstruction	Upper airway irritation symptoms Vocal cord dysfunction
RADS	Irritant-induced asthma
Adult respiratory distress syndrome	Bronchiolitis obliterans (popcorn lung)
Bronchiolitis obliterans	Decrease in spirometric tests Increased airway hyperresponsiveness Enhanced cough reflex Potentiating of allergen effect Increased exhaled-breath nitric oxide Induced sputum neutrophilia

Approximately 6% to 22% of the cases of occupational asthma are considered irritant-induced.[25,28,30,31] Most cases of occupational asthma are attributed to allergic sensitization. A retrospective study of 469 asthma claims accepted by the Ontario Workers' Compensation Board between 1984 and 1988 identified 89 people (19%) who developed asthma after a accidental high irritant exposure (ie, RADS), 68 people (76%) who reportedly had an exacerbation of preexisting asthma, and 12 people (13%) who claimed new-onset irritant-induced asthma.[32] Data from a Chinese community-based study of 3606 adults report the adjusted attributable risk for asthma due to irritant gases or fumes to be 1.2%.[33]

RADS

Some inhalation events hold serious consequences. There may be corneal and nasal mucosal damage if the face is involved. Upper airway localization may cause swelling of the tongue, persistent rhinitis, or closure of the glottis and larynx.[34] More distal damage can lead to adult respiratory distress syndrome (ARDS) or persistent bronchiolar obstruction (bronchiolitis obliterans). Some inhalation injuries lead to acute irritant-induced asthma (RADS).[23,35–37] **Box 1** presents the diagnostic criteria for RADS.[35]

The denotation, RADS, applies to events in which onset of acute asthma follows exposure to a single high-level irritant gas, vapor, or fume. The asthmatic process proceeds without latency or immunologic sensitization.

Box 1 Diagnostic criteria for RADS
1. Absence of preexisting respiratory disorder, asthma symptoms, or a history of asthma in remission; and exclusion of conditions that can simulate asthma
2. Onset of asthma after a single exposure or accident
3. Exposure is to irritant vapor, gas, fumes, or smoke in very high concentrations
4. Onset of asthma occurs within minutes to hours and always less than 24 hours after the exposure
5. Finding of a positive methacholine challenge test (<8 mg/mL) following the exposure
6. Possible airflow obstruction on pulmonary function testing
7. Another pulmonary disorder to explain the symptoms and findings is excluded.

Almost all instances of RADS are accidental and it is not possible to quantify the exact magnitude of the emitted irritant exposure causing RADS. Typically, the exposure is caused by an explosion, accidental release of irritants under pressure, or a reduced ventilation exchange rate (as in a confined space). The exposure consists of a vapor, gas, fume, or smoke. High-level dust exposures are rarely the cause. In the authors' opinion, the designation of RADS for rescue works involved in the collapse of the World Trade Center is questionable.[38]

Most persons are overwhelmed by the exposure and require immediate medical attention. On examination, these individuals demonstrate clinical findings that support the presence of a serious inhalation injury. The hallmark of RADS is persistent, nonspecific, airway hyperresponsiveness. At time of medical examination, subjects show a positive methacholine challenge test with provocative concentration of methacholine causing a 20% fall in forced expiratory volume in one second (PC_{20}) of less than or equal to 8 mg/mL. Patients have negative chest radiographs. Pulmonary function tests are normal or show mild airflow limitation. Significant persistent airflow limitation occurs only in a small percentage of persons with RADS. It is important that, other pulmonary diseases be eliminated. Following the exposure, most persons with RADS take antiasthma medications that they were not taking before the exposure.

The criteria for diagnosing RADS is secure (ie, single and high-level exposure) but there is a reluctance in accepting alternative types of irritant-induced asthma; for instance, in cases of low-dose or repeated (days, weeks, months) exposures to irritant gases, vapors, or fumes.[31,39] The diagnostic criteria for RADS promulgated by the Workers Compensation System in South Africa require all of the following five findings[40]: (1) history indicating the absence of preexisting asthma-like complaints; (2) onset of symptoms after single or multiple exposures, incidents, or accidents; (3) occupational exposure to a gas, smoke, fume, vapor, or dust with irritant properties; (4) onset of symptoms within 24 hours of exposure, with persistence of symptoms for at least 3 months (there must be an association between symptoms of asthma and exposure); and (5) presence of airflow obstruction on pulmonary function tests and/ or presence of nonspecific bronchial hyperresponsiveness on tests done at least 3 months after exposure. These diagnostic criteria are similar to the ones mentioned in the original description of the disorder (see **Box 1**).[35]

An early contention is that multiple exposures to low concentrations of an irritant chemical can lead to a RADS-like picture (ie, low-dose RADS).[41] The designation of low-dose RADS, with a background of repeated low-dose (as opposed to a single high-dose) exposure, is controversial and not generally accepted.[23,25,27,42–44]

There continues to be a controversy concerning the pathophysiology of RADS. It is not known whether host susceptibility factors (eg, cigarette smoking, genetic predisposition, preexisting lung disease, or atopy) are prerequisites for RADS development. Alternatively, an atopic-type person may predispose to non-RADS, irritant-induced asthma.[24,26,45–47] Brooks[24] hypothesizes that other than established RADS, countless designations of irritant-induced asthma (including low-dose RADS) are actually an exacerbation of asthma among persons with preexisting asthma in remission or persons manifesting relatively mild or asymptomatic asthma not requiring medications (asymptomatic airway hyperresponsiveness).[24,48,49]

Causes of RADS

The originally reported causes of RADS include uranium hexafluoride gas, floor sealant, spray paint containing significant concentrations of ammonia, heated acid, 35-percent hydrazine, fumigating fog, metal coating remover, and smoke.[35] Other reported examples of RADS include sulfuric acid or SO_2; smoke inhalation; locomotive or diesel exhaust; hydrochloric acid; floor sealant; anhydrous ammonia fumes; silo gas; acetic acid; burned paint fumes; zinc chloride; chlorine gas; welding fumes; phosphoric acid or disinfectant; phosgene; anticorrosive agent (2-diethylaminoethanolamine); bleaching agents; constituent of free-base cocaine; sodium hydroxide, silicon tetrachloride, or trichlorosilane exposure; burning paint fumes; toluene diisocyanate; metam sodium pesticide environmental spill; irritant gas containing chromate; nonspecified irritants; and tear gas.[25,30,50] Kern[51] noted a dose–response relationship for RADS development occurring among hospital workers exposed to a spill of 100% glacial acetic acid. Those subjects with RADS seemed to have suffered the higher dose exposures and were closer to the spill. RADS resolved in some subjects and, in others, RADS manifestations persisted for nearly a year after the accident. **Table 2** summarizes outcomes from a single or repeated irritant exposure.

Natural History of RADS

The prognosis for RADS is variable and the determining factors are unclear. Symptoms can be transient and resolve in less than 12 weeks. Conversely, in some patients, symptoms may persist for many years.[28] One review of RADS cases reported a median duration of symptoms lasting 13 months (interquartile range, 6.5–43.5 months).[52] In a study by Malo and colleagues,[28] about 35% of patients reported persistent asthma-like symptoms, about one-third of the subjects were using inhaled corticosteroids, and one-third of participants were still smoking. More than 50% of participants noted continued asthmatic symptoms for years after their inhalational accident and more than one-third showed persistent nonspecific airway hyperresponsiveness. Subjects reported high levels of anxiety and depression. Individuals demonstrating functional improvement tended to be younger and show a higher baseline methacholine PC_{20}. Being younger may represent a positive prognostic feature.[53]

The type of causal agent (chlorine gas vs others), the interval since the accident, and a visit to an emergency room or hospitalization did not influence the prognosis.[28] Cigarette smoking may play an additive role because smokers showed poorer pulmonary function tests at follow-up evaluations. Gautrin and colleagues[54] noted that both cigarette smoking and the number of "puffs" of chlorine (ie, the occurrence of symptoms that did not result in visits to a first-aid unit) applied a significant additive effect on the reduction in lung function tests and on methacholine hyperresponsiveness over time.

Overall, workplace inhalation accidents have a good prognosis. They are especially common in the chemical, plastics, and engineering sectors. About 10% of patients report persistent respiratory symptoms among 383 inhalation accidents in a study from the United Kingdom. Only 3% of patients showed persistent asthma.[55]

NONASTHMA AIRWAY CHANGES CAUSED BY IRRITANTS
Breathing-Pattern Changes

Purportedly, sensory irritants stimulate nasal trigeminal C fibers to decrease the breathing rate by inducing a prolonged pause at the start of expiration.[56–59] The potency of a sensory irritant has been quantified by determining the concentration of the irritant that produces a 50% decrease in breathing rate (RD_{50}) of rodents (especially mice).[56]

Reduction in Forced Expiratory Volume in One Second

Gautrin and colleagues[60] assessed 239 workers in a metal processing plant who experienced repeated exposures to chlorine gas as documented by first-aid records and a detailed occupational history on the occurrence of chlorine puffs. There was reduction in forced expiratory volume in one second (FEV_1), especially in symptomatic workers. In a subsequent 2-year follow-up study, a decrease in lung function was associated with chlorine gassing incidents; the numbers of chlorine puffs caused mild symptoms mainly among cigarette smokers of 20 packs per year or more.[54] Another study confirmed that 13 of 278 workers reported a gassing incident to the first aid unit. Three of these 13 workers showed normal baseline spirometry and bronchial responsiveness. Subsequently, there were transient but significant changes in lung-function testing.[61]

Enhanced Airway Responsiveness

Enhanced methacholine responsiveness, determined by dose response slope and detectable increase in airway responsiveness (PC_{20} decrease $\geq$1.5-fold), was associated with chlorine gassing events.[54,60] Another study of 20 pulp mill workers experiencing repeated chlorine gas exposures showed airway hyperresponsiveness when first assessed.[62] There was a follow-up study of these workers who repeatedly inhaled puffs of high concentrations of chlorine over a 3-month period. Although spirometry changes persisted, bronchial hyperresponsiveness improved significantly in those with normal airway caliber, suggesting that less pronounced bronchial alterations induced by repeated exposures to chlorine might be reversible.

Potentiating or Adjuvant Effect of an Allergen

Preexposure to permissible concentrations of air pollutants, such as SO_2, ozone, and nitrogen dioxide, leads to an enhanced airway response to the allergen.[18,63,64] In allergen-challenge studies of adults with mild allergic asthma, initial ozone exposure enhances the specific bronchial response to the allergen and potentiates the subsequent eosinophilic inflammation.[64,65] The mechanism is unknown but in some manner, there is priming of the airway mucosa and enhancement of the cellular responses to allergen and evolution of airway inflammation.[66] Thus, persons with previous allergies become "primed" or "potentiated" after an irritant exposure and now react to lower concentrations of the allergen to which they previously did not react.

Inflammatory Changes—Identified by Noninvasive Approaches

A variety of respiratory diseases have been explored measuring constituents present in exhaled breath gas (eg, exhaled breath nitric oxide [E_{NO}]) and exhaled breath condensate.[67] E_{NO} may reflect airway inflammation in workers with exposure to elevated concentrations of ozone. Pulp-mill workers reporting ozone-gassing incidents demonstrated elevated E_{NO} levels.[68,69] Increased levels of E_{NO} were apparent in a group of underground workers with exposure to particulates and nitrogen dioxide when compared with outdoor workers who cut concrete.[70] E_{NO} levels increased 40% at the end of shift from a pre-exposure level in a group of shoe and leather workers having exposure to toluene, xylene, and methyl ethyl ketone.[71] Sputum analysis provides another noninvasive method of examining the airway secretions of subjects with asthma. Sputum cellular responses in asthma may show either eosinophilic or neutrophilic patterns.[72–74] Cases of proclaimed irritant-induced asthma show increase numbers of neutrophils in the induced sputum after paint fumes, grain dust, and ozone exposures.[75]

Irritant-Induced Cough

Repeated and/or prolonged inhalational exposures to various irritating gases, vapors, dusts, and fumes lead to the development of chronic cough.[23,76–83] Symptomatic glass bottle workers chronically exposed to a variety of workplace irritants, including hydrochloric acid aerosol, report a higher prevalence of nose and throat irritation complaints, and cough progressing to shortness of breath.[84,85] In a laboratory setting, greater cough sensitivity to citric acid and capsaicin aerosols is observed in symptomatic workers. The latent interval between starting work and first developing symptoms is typically 4 years. Blanc and colleagues[86] report that chili pepper workers continually exposed to capsaicin experience chronic cough.

POTENTIAL PATHOGENETIC MECHANISMS TO EXPLAIN IRRITANT EFFECTS

With RADS, the respiratory tract reacts to a massive irritant exposure with a constellation of cellular and biochemical proceedings. Subsequent nonimmunologic processes, such as mononuclear cell infiltrate and edema are key components in RADS development. Pathologic findings from the original report of RADS show epithelial cellular injury, bronchial wall inflammation, and lymphocytes and plasma cells infiltration without eosinophilia.[35] There is no evidence of mucous gland hyperplasia, basement membrane thickening, or smooth muscle hypertrophy.

Cough is a common complaint of RADS patients. Persons with chronic cough not associated with asthma manifest airway inflammation that is distinctly different from the inflammation noted among asthmatic individuals with persistent cough.[87] For the nonasthmatics with cough, there are increases in the numbers of submucosal mast cells (but not neutrophils or eosinophils). Additionally, there is airway wall remodeling with goblet cell hyperplasia, subepithelial fibrosis, increase in airway smooth muscle cells, and increased vascularity.[87] Perhaps, airway wall remodeling after an irritant exposure is due to a tissue repair response to injury. Irritant-induced inflammatory damage or derangement may target the epithelial-mesenchymal unit.[88] Investigations that examined biopsied bronchial tissue obtained shortly after a high-level irritant exposure reveal rapid denudation of the bronchial mucosal surface with submucosal fibrohemorrhagic exudates and subepithelial edema.[89] The airway mucosa regenerates from proliferating basal and parabasalar cells over the subsequent several months.

Following airway epithelial damage, the airway epithelium promptly reestablishes an epithelial sheet with normal structure and function.[90] The cells of the normal airway epithelium turn over every 30 to 50 days. Supposedly, the bronchial epithelium regenerates itself through a GATA binding protein 6 (Gata6) mechanisms and activation of endogenous stem cells.[91] Gata6-regulated Wnt signaling controls the balance between progenitor expansion and epithelial differentiation necessary for lung regeneration.[91]

It seems that airway remodeling leads to persistent structural changes, chronic airway inflammation, and continual airway hyperresponsiveness.[92–94] During normal circumstances, injury to the airway epithelium stimulates the intrinsic repair pathway with healing by primary intention. Possibly, in RADS, there is an impaired airway repair response to injury that mimics the chronic wound scenario of healing by secondary intention.[95] This hypothetical scenario likely requires a genetic susceptibility.

Special airway nociceptors nestled within nerve fibers express dozens of ion channels that detect noxious stimuli.[12,13,96,97] The transient receptor potential vanilloid-1 (TRPV$_1$) and transient receptor potential cation channel, subfamily A, member 1 (TRPA$_1$) are two types (and perhaps there are more) of ion channel proteins of particular interest.[98,99] The TRPV$_1$ is activated by capsaicin and other vanilloids; moderate noxious heat ($\geq$42°C); low pH ($\leq$5.9), and a host of inflammatory mediators.[100–105] Greater TRPV$_1$ activity has been linked to chronic cough.[106,107] The TRPA$_1$, another excitatory ion channel, has been referred to as the irritant receptor and possibly provides the transduction mechanism through which environmental irritants depolarize lung nociceptors to elicit responses.[108–110] Stimulation of the $TRPA_1$ receptor also induces cough. The $TRPA_1$ channel is activated by a wide range of irritant chemicals including acrolein, horseradish, menthol, formalin, garlic, and others.[100,110–112]

Although unproven, the mechanism to explain irritant-induced asthma with nonspecific airway hyperresponsiveness (as seen in RADS) may be from heightened responsiveness of the $TRPV_1$ and $TRPA_1$ channels.[113] Perhaps, severe inhalational, irritant-induced, airways damage causes chronic airways inflammation, a rejoinder to the release of tissue injury and inflammatory products (eg, bradykinin, ATP, prostaglandin E_2, nerve growth factor, proteases, serotonin).[114,115] In a sustained and potentiated state, $TRPV_1$ and $TRPA_1$ channels manifest much higher neuronal Ca^{2+} responsiveness to the irritant chemicals and there is recruitment of other neurons previously not responsive. In this state of heightened $TRPV_1$ and $TRPA_1$ sensitivity, both noxious and innocuous stimuli produce exaggerated or prolonged biochemical and physiologic effects.[96] Furthermore, there may be greater release of neuropeptides from the neuronal terminals leading to neurogenic inflammation.[116–120] Nervous tissue growth and neural plasticity may translate as bronchial hyperresponsiveness, a characteristic of irritant-induced asthma.[117,121–129]

IRRITANT-INDUCED ASTHMA: GENUINE AND MOCK
Cleaning Materials

Studies conducted in several countries report higher risks for asthma among professional cleaners experiencing repeated exposures to many irritating chemicals, such as bleach, aerosol disinfectants, and cleaning agents.[130–132] A surveillance study in California (1993–1996) reports janitors and cleaners have the highest average annual rate of work-related asthma.[133] National Health and Nutrition Examination Survey (NHANES) III data show cleaners have the fourth highest odds ratio (OR = 5.44, 95% CI 2.43–12.18) for work-related wheeze among 28 occupational categories.[134] The European Community Respiratory Health Survey (ECRHS) concludes cleaners display the fourth highest odds ratio for asthma (OR = 1.97, 95% CI 1.33–2.92) among 29 occupational groups.[135]

World Trade Center Illnesses

On September 11, 2001, the destruction and collapse of the World Trade Center towers generated an intense, short-term exposure to inorganic dust, pyrolysis products, and other respirable materials. Firefighters and other rescue workers were exposed to the high levels of the dust and other particulate materials especially during the first few days after the World Trade Center collapse.[136] The composition of the dust was highly alkaline and contained up to 2% respirable particulate matter.[136–138] Following the World Trade Center collapse, several respiratory illnesses were described among rescue workers, including what has been called World Trade Center cough, persistent hyperreactivity, RADS, and acute eosinophilic pneumonia.[136,139,140] As mentioned, the designation of RADS for rescue works involved in the collapse of the World Trade Center has been called into question.[38]

Ozone

The ozone response can be summarized as (1) cough and chest pain worsened by deep inspiration[141]; (2) declines in forced vital capacity (FVC) and FEV_1 thought to result from involuntary inhibition of full inspiration[142]; (3) greater responsiveness to ozone by young than older persons[143–145]; (4) changes in the breathing pattern (increased respiratory rate and tidal ventilation)[146]; (5) attenuation of pulmonary responses after repeated ozone exposures[63,147]; (6) introduction of bronchoalveolar lavage neutrophilia, protein leakage, and presence of proinflammatory cytokines after ozone inhalation[148–151]; (7) transient increase in nonspecific bronchial hyperresponsiveness in normal and asthmatic subjects; and (8) enhanced response to allergen challenge among asthmatic subjects breathing ozone.[144,152] Although ozone inhalation manifests prominent irritation properties, there are individual variability of responses.

Asthma-Like Symptoms and Odor

Perhaps 15% to 30% of the general population asserts increased sensitivity to chemicals in their environment.[153–155] The term airway sensory hyperreactivity applies to patients with upper and lower airway complaints induced by scents and inhaled chemicals such as perfumes, flowers, colored paints, cigarette smoke, and automobile exhaust fumes.[156] These individuals show increased cough sensitivity by capsaicin-challenge testing, and poorer quality of life scores but no greater sensitivity to methacholine.[157,158] The interpretation of these studies is limited by the small subject population size, lack of customary standards for administration of cough challenges, and virtually no assessment of environmental or occupational exposures.[156,157,159] There is also controversy with those investigations using the uncertain term chemical sensitivity to explain a condition based solely on self-reporting of symptoms and a perceived exposure recognized principally by an odor. Overall, qualitative estimates of chemical sensitivity based solely on reports of illness caused by odors have little validity.

Potroom Asthma

Potroom asthma applies to the asthma-like syndrome that afflicts workers employed in the production of aluminum smelting, where the alumina is partially dissolved in an electrolyte of molten cryolite at about 960°C.[160,161] A dose–response relationship has been described for fluoride exposure and airway hyperresponsiveness in potroom workers.[162] However, the role of fluorides as causative agents, coagents, or markers for the causative agents of potroom asthma is undetermined. There has been documentation of a dual asthmatic reaction with an associated increase in nonspecific airway responsiveness after exposure to the potroom workplace.[163] Bronchial biopsies obtained in workers with potroom asthma show pathologic alterations similar to those described in other types of asthma.

Eosinophilic Bronchitis

Eosinophilic bronchitis is a term relegated to a group of patients with chronic cough, sputum eosinophilia, normal spirometry, absence of airway hyperresponsiveness, and normal peak expiratory flow variability.[3,164] These patients do not meet the conventional criteria for the diagnosis of asthma. There is subjective improvement in cough and a significant decrease in sputum eosinophil count after treatment with inhaled corticosteroids.[165,166] The clinical presentation has been reported in workers exposed to acrylates, latex, mushroom spores, and lysozymes.[167]

Vocal Cord Dysfunction

Vocal cord closure on inspiration causes airflow obstruction, wheezing, and occasionally stridor. The manifestation of vocal cord dysfunction (VCD) presents during inspiration but may persist into expiration. About 10% of patients referred for refractory asthma have a diagnosis of VCD. An additional 33% have VCD accompanying asthma. There are more women with a diagnosis of VCD. Unlike asthmatics, VCD patients rarely awaken from sleep by attacks. Psychogenic factors are believed to contribute to cases of VCD. Irritants, such as dust, smoke, chemicals, and odors may precipitate attacks in VCD patients. Perkner and colleagues[168] reported on 11 cases of VCD in which there was a temporal association between VCD onset and occupational or environmental irritant exposure. Huggins and colleagues[169] studied a 46-year-old woman with VCD precipitated by eucalyptus exposure. A definitive VCD diagnosis requires visualization of the vocal cords via laryngoscopy.[170] Typically, VCD appears as adduction of the anterior two-thirds of the vocal cords with posterior chinking that creates a diamond shape. Both exercise and methacholine challenge can induce symptoms in patients with VCD. Speech therapy is the first line of treatment for VCD and may be sufficient to correct the disorder. Therapy involves techniques emphasizing decreasing laryngeal muscle tone, largely by helping patients focus on expiration instead of inspiration. Bronchodilator inhalers and corticosteroids used to treat asthma are not effective.

Meat Wrapper's Asthma

In 1973, three workers employed as meat wrappers developed respiratory symptoms after exposure to fumes of polyvinyl chloride film cut with a hot wire.[171] The name of the syndrome is meat wrapper's asthma. Subsequently, there were several other reports of patients with diverse symptoms, including rhinorrhea, cough, tightness of the chest, sore throat, exhaustion, wheezing, and throat soreness. Some investigators conclude that the emission from thermally activated price labels is the principal cause of meat wrapper's asthma. Subsequent investigations fail to confirm that any major airways condition affects meat wrappers and designation of asthma is a misnomer.[172]

Pesticides

There are studies, describing an association between risk for asthma and pesticide aerial spraying, application or exposure in a variety of populations.[173,174] Cone and colleagues[175] describe asthma after metam sodium pesticide spill.

Formaldehyde

Most respiratory complaints from formaldehyde are due to its irritant nature.[176,177] There is a report of asthma developing in pathologists and nurses working in a dialysis unit exposed to high levels of formaldehyde.[178]

Cotton and Textiles

The spectrum of byssinosis ranges from acute dyspnea and chest tightness on 1 or more days of a workweek (ie, acute byssinosis) to a permanent obstructive airways disease.[179] Atopy may act as a risk factor for the airway response to cotton dust. The prevalence of the symptoms is associated with the magnitude of the cotton dust level and, especially, the coarse protein particles rather than the mineral or cellulose portion of the cotton. Airway responses also occur after exposures to the dusts of flax, jute, sisal, or soft hemp. Mechanisms to explain byssinosis include the direct mediator release from mast cells following inhalation of the dust; an endotoxin-like action of the dust from gram-negative bacterial (mainly *Enterobacter*) contamination of the cotton; or, unlikely, an allergic mechanism. The exact role of cigarette smoking for the chronic form of the disease is unclear.

Red-Tide Toxin

A natural phenomenon caused by the blooms of the unicellular marine alga *Ptychodiscus brevis* occurs in the Gulf of Mexico, mainly along the west coast of Florida. Red tide is reported to produce asthma-like symptoms in humans and contraction in vitro of canine airway smooth muscle preparations.[180]

Machining Fluids

The exact ingredient of machining fluids responsible for the acute FEV_1 changes is not clear, but there have been reports of asthma due to additives of machining fluids.[181,182] It is speculated that microbial contaminations with endotoxin from gram-negative bacteria or chemical irritant additives are potential causes.

Bronchiolitis Obliterans

Bronchiolitis obliterans evolves after inhaling an irritant gas, fume, or vapor (and rarely dust), such as nitrogen dioxide, sulfur dioxide, ammonia, chlorine, phosgene, hot gases, or fly ash.[37,183–186] There are sporadic cases of bronchiolitis obliterans among nylon-flock workers, workers who spray prints onto textiles using polyamide-amine dyes, battery workers (who are exposed to thionyl chloride fumes), and workers in the food-flavoring industry.[187] Bronchiolitis obliterans has been reported among microwave popcorn production workers who developed cough, shortness of breath, and wheezing 5 months to 9 years after starting work at the popcorn plant.[188,189] Butter flavoring vapors containing 203 to 371 ppm diacetyl caused necrotizing and suppurative changes of four levels of the rat's nose.[190] A cross-sectional evaluation of 117 current workers conducted by Kreiss and colleagues[191] showed a strong relation between the quartile of estimated cumulative exposure to diacetyl and the frequency and extent of airway obstruction.

SUMMARY

There are many unanswered questions concerning the pathogenesis of RADS and irritancy. A limited numbers of studies address the long-term prognosis of RADS. Do genetic factors play a role in RADS development? If so, what host factors are requisite for developing irritant-induced asthma? What role do ion channels play in RADS development and asthma in general? Understanding basic issues regarding irritancy and irritant-induced asthma may lead to therapeutic options to improve treatment of these disorders.

REFERENCES

1. Newman-Taylor A, Cullinan P, Burge PS, et al. BOHRF guidelines for occupational asthma. Thorax 2005;60:364–6.
2. Francis HC, Prys-Picard CO, Fishwick D, et al. Defining and investigating occupational asthma: a consensus approach. Occup Environ Med 2007;64:361–5.
3. Tarlo SM, Balmes J, Balkissoon R, et al. Diagnosis and management of work-related asthma. American College of Chest Physicians Consensus Statement. Chest 2008;134(3):1S–41S.
4. Goe S, Henneberger P, Reilly M, et al. A descriptive study of work aggravated asthma. Occup Environ Med 2004;61:512–7.
5. Saarinen K, Karjalainen A, Martikainen R, et al. Prevalence of work-aggravated symptoms in clinically established asthma. Eur Respir J 2003;22:305–9.

6. Blanc PD, Galbo M, Hiatt P, et al. Morbidity following acute irritant inhalation in a population based study. JAMA 1991;266:664–9.

7. Henneberger PK, Metayer C, Layne LA, et al. Nonfatal work-related inhalations: surveillance data from hospital emergency departments, 1995-1996. Am J Ind Med 2000;38:140–8.

8. Wesselkamper SC, Prows DR, Biswas P, et al. Genetic susceptibility to irritant-induced acute lung injury in mice. Am J Physiol Lung Cell Mol Physiol 2000; 279:L575–82.

9. Leikauf GD, McDowell SA, Wesselkamper SC, et al. Acute lung injury. Functional genomics and genetic susceptibility. Chest 2002;121:70S–5S.

10. Occupational Safety and Health Administration (OSHA): OSHA Hazard Communication Standard (HCS) in 29 CFR 19101200 (Department of Labor Vol. Appendix A to the Hazard Communication Standard, 29 CFR 1910.1200). Washington, DC: OSHA; 1994.

11. Safety and Environment Unit. Glossary of Chemical Terms. 2007. Available at: http://www.Weizmann.ac.IL/Safety/chgl.html. Accessed September 20, 2007.

12. Cometto Muniz JE, Cain WS, Abraham MH, et al. Chemical boundaries for detection of eye irritation in humans from homologous vapors. Toxicol Sci 2006;9:600–9.

13. Ferrer Montiel A, Garcia Martinez C, Morenilla Palao C, et al. Molecular architecture of the vanilloid receptor. Insights for drug design. Eur J Biochem 2004;271: 1820–6.

14. Blum E, Liu K, Mazourek M, et al. Molecular mapping of the C locus for presence of pungency in Capsicum. Genome 2002;45:702–5.

15. Prasad BC, Kumar V, Gururaj HB, et al. Characterization of capsaicin synthase and identification of its gene (CSY 1) for pungency factor capsaicin in pepper (capsicum SP.). Proc Natl Acad Sci U S A 2006;103:13315–20.

16. Randle W, Bussard ML. Streamlining onion pungency analyses. HortScience 1993;28:60.

17. Cometto-Muftiz JE, Cain WS. Relative sensitivity of the ocular trigeminal, nasal trigeminal and olfactory systems to airborne chemicals. Chem Senses 1995; 20(2):191–8.

18. Molfino N, Wright S, Katz I, et al. Effect of low concentrations of ozone on inhaled allergen responses in asthmatic subjects. Lancet 1991;338:199–203.

19. King C, Brennan S, Thompson PJ, et al. Dust mite proteolytic allergens induce cytokine release from cultured airway epithelium. J Immunol 1998;161:3645–51.

20. Kato A, Favoreto JS, Avila PC, et al. TLR-3-and Th-2 cytokine dependent production of thymic stromal lymphopoietin in human airway epithelial cells. J Immunol 2007;179:1080–7.

21. Stedman's Medical Dictionary. Online Medical Dictionary. 2007. 27th edition. Available at: http://www.stedmans.com/Section.cfm/45. Accessed September 22, 2007.

22. Shusterman D. Sequelae of respiratory tract exposures to irritant chemicals. Pulmonary and critical care update. American College of Chest Physicians 2001;15(Lesson 2):1–4. Available at: http://chestnet.org/education/online/pccu/vol15/lessons1_2/lesson02.php. Accessed July 26, 2011.

23. Brooks SM. Inhalation airway injury: a spectrum of changes. Clin Pulm Med 2007;14:1–8.

24. Brooks SM, Hammad Y, Richards I, et al. The spectrum of irritant induced asthma: sudden and not so sudden onset and the role of allergy. Chest 1998; 113(1):42–9.

25. Gautrin D, Bernstein IL, Brooks SM, et al. Reactive airways dysfunction syndrome or irritant induced asthma. In: Bernstein DI, Chan-Yeung M, Malo J-L, et al, editors. Asthma in the workplace and related conditions. 3rd edition. New York: Taylor and Francis; 2006. p. 581–629.

26. Mapp CE, Boschetto P, Maestrelli P, et al. Occupational asthma: state of the art. Am J Respir Crit Care Med 2005;172:288–305.

27. Lemière C, Malo JL, Gautrin D. Nonsensitizing causes of occupational asthma. Med Clin North Am 1996;80(4):749–74.

28. Malo JL, L'archeveque J, Castellanos L, et al. Long-term outcomes of acute irritant induced asthma. Am J Respir Crit Care Med 2009;179:923–8.

29. Cullinan P, Acquilla S, Dhara VR. Respiratory morbidity 10 years after the union carbide gas leak at Bhopal: a cross sectional survey. BMJ 1997;314:338–42.

30. Brooks SM, Truncale T, McCluskey J. Occupational and environmental asthma. In: Rom WM, editor. Environmental and occupational medicine. Lippincott Raven Publishers; 2007. p. 418–63.

31. Tarlo SM. Workplace irritant exposures: do they produce true occupational asthma? Ann Allergy Asthma Immunol 2003;90(5 Suppl 2):19–23.

32. Chatkin JM, Tarlo SM, Liss G, et al. The outcome of asthma related to workplace irritant exposures: a comparison of irritant induced asthma and irritant aggravation of asthma. Chest 1999;116:1780–5.

33. Xu X, Christiani DC. Occupational exposures and physician diagnosed asthma. Chest 1993;104(5):1364–70.

34. Shusterman D. Review of the upper airway, including olfaction, as mediator of symptoms. Environ Health Perspect 2002;4:649–53.

35. Brooks SM, Weiss MA, Bernstein IL. Reactive airways dysfunction syndrome (RADS). Persistent asthma syndrome after high level irritant exposures. Chest 1985;88(3):376–84.

36. Meggs WV, Cleveland CH, Metger WJ, et al. Reactive upper airway dysfunction syndrome (RUDS): a form of irritant rhinitis induced by chemical exposure. J Allergy Clin Immunol 1992;89:170.

37. Schachter EN, Zuskin E, Saric M. Occupational airway diseases. Rev Environ Health 2001;16(2):87–95.

38. Truncale T, Brooks SM. World Trade Center dust and airway reactivity (letter to the editor). Am J Respir Crit Care Med 2004;169:883–5.

39. Gautrin D, Bernstein IL, Brooks SM. Reactive airways dysfunction syndrome, or irritant induced asthma. Edition. In: Bernstein IL, Chan-Yeung M, Luc Malo J, et al, editors. Asthma in the workplace. New York: Marcel Dekker, Inc; 1999. p. 565–93.

40. Jeebhay A, Quirce S. Occupational asthma in the developing and industrialized world: a review. Int J Tuberc Lung Dis 2007;11:122–33.

41. Kipen HM, Blume R, Hutt D. Asthma experience in an occupational and environmental medicine clinic. Low-dose reactive airways dysfunction syndrome [See Comments]. J Occup Med 1994;36(10):1133–7.

42. Malo JL. Irritant induced asthma and reactive airways dysfunction syndrome. Can Respir J 1998;5(1):66–7.

43. Tarlo S, Boulet LP, Cartier A, et al. Canadian thoracic society guidelines for occupational asthma. Can Respir J 1998;4:289–300.

44. Tarlo SM, Liss GM. Evidence based guidelines for the prevention, identification, and management of occupational asthma. Occup Environ Med 2005;62(5):288–9.

45. Medina-Ramón M, Zock JP, Kogevinas M, et al. Asthma, chronic bronchitis, and exposure to irritant agents in occupational domestic cleaning: a nested case-control study. Occup Environ Med 2005;62:598–606.

46. Tarlo SM, Broder I. Irritant induced occupational asthma. Chest 1989;96(2): 297–300.
47. Vandenplas O, Malo JL. Definitions and types of work-related asthma: a nosological approach. Eur Respir J 2003;21(4):706–12.
48. Boulet LP. Asymptomatic airway hyperresponsiveness. Am J Respir Crit Care Med 2003;167:371–8.
49. Laprise C, Boulet LP. Asymptomatic airway hyperresponsiveness: a three-year follow-up. Am J Respir Crit Care Med 1997;156:403–9.
50. Alberts WM, Do Pico GA. Reactive airways dysfunction syndrome. Chest 1996; 109(6):1618–26.
51. Kern DG. Outbreak of the reactive airways dysfunction syndrome after a spill of glacial acetic. Am Rev Respir Dis 1991;144:1058–64.
52. Shakeri MS, Dick FD, Ayres JG. Which agents cause reactive airways dysfunction syndrome (RADS)? A systematic review. Occup Med (Lond) 2008;58:205–11.
53. Rachiotis G, Savani R, Brant A, et al. Outcome of occupational asthma after cessation of exposure: a systematic review. Thorax 2007;62:147–52.
54. Gautrin D, Leroyer C, Infante-Rivard C, et al. Longitudinal assessment of airway caliber and responsiveness in workers exposed to chlorine. Am J Respir Crit Care Med 1999;160:1232–7.
55. Sallie B, Mcdonald C. Inhalation accidents reported to the sword surveillance project 1990-1993. Ann Occup Hyg 1996;40(2):211–21.
56. Alarie Y. Sensory irritation by airborne chemicals. CRC Crit Rev Toxicol 1973;3: 299–363.
57. Morris JB, Symanowicz PT, Olsen JE, et al. Immediate sensory nerve-mediated respiratory responses to irritants in healthy and allergic airway-diseased mice. J Appl Physiol 2003;94:1563–71.
58. Gagnaire F, Marignac B, Morel G, et al. Sensory irritation due to methyl-2-cyanoacrylate, ethyl-2-cyanoacrylate, isopropyl-2-cyanoacrylate and 2-methoxyethyl-2-cyanoacrylate in mice. Ann Occup Hyg 2003;47:297–304.
59. Gagnaire F, Marignac B, Hecht G, et al. Sensory irritation of acetic acid, hydrogen peroxide, peroxyacetic acid and their mixture in mice. Ann Occup Hyg 2001;46:97–102.
60. Gautrin D, Leroyer C, L'archeveque J, et al. Cross-sectional assessment of workers with repeated exposure to chlorine over a three year period. Eur Respir J 1995;8(12):2046–54.
61. Leroyer C, Malo JL, Infante-Rivard C, et al. Changes in airway function and bronchial responsiveness after acute occupational exposure to chlorine leading to treatment in a first aid unit. Occup Environ Med 1998;55(5):356–9.
62. Malo JL, Cartier A, Boulet LP, et al. Bronchial hyperresponsiveness can improve while spirometry plateaus two to three years after repeated exposure to chlorine causing respiratory symptoms. Am J Respir Crit Care Med 1994;150(4):1142–5.
63. Jorres R, Nowak D, Magnussen H, et al. The effect of ozone exposure on allergen responsiveness in subjects with asthma or rhinitis. Short-term O3 increases bronchial allergen response with mild allergic asthma or rhinitis without asthma. Am J Respir Crit Care Med 1996;153:56–64.
64. Osebold J, Gershwin L, Zee Y. Studies on the enhancement of allergic sensitization by the inhalation of ozone and sulfuric acid aerosol. J Environ Pathol Toxicol Oncol 1990;3:221–34.
65. Vagaggini B, Taccola M, Cianchetti S, et al. Ozone exposure increases eosinophilic airway response induced by previous allergen challenge. Am J Respir Crit Care Med 2002;166:1073–7.

66. Peden DB, Setzer RW Jr, Devlin RB. Ozone exposure has both a priming effect on allergen-induced responses and an intrinsic inflammatory action in the nasal airways of perennially allergic asthmatics. Am J Respir Crit Care Med 1995; 151(5):1336–45.

67. Kharitonov SA, Barnes PJ. Exhaled markers of pulmonary disease. Am J Respir Crit Care Med 2001;163(7):1693–722.

68. Olin A, Ljungkvist G, Bake B, et al. Exhaled nitric oxide among pulpmill workers reporting gassing incidents involving ozone and chlorine dioxide. Eur Respir J 1999;14(4):828–31.

69. Olin AC, Andersson E, Andersson M, et al. Prevalence of asthma and exhaled nitric oxide are increased in bleachery workers exposed to ozone. Eur Respir J 2004;23(1):87–92.

70. Ulvestad B, Lund MB, Bakke B, et al. Gas and dust exposure in underground construction is associated with signs of airway inflammation. Eur Respir J 2001;17(3):416–21.

71. Maniscalco M, Grieco L, Galdi A, et al. Increase in exhaled nitric oxide in shoe and leather workers at the end of the work-shift. Occup Med (Lond) 2004;54(6):404–7.

72. Douwes J, Gibson P, Pekkanen J, et al. Non-eosinophilic asthma: importance and possible mechanisms. Thorax 2002;57(7):643–8.

73. Simpson JL, Wood LG, Gibson PG. Inflammatory mediators in exhaled breath, induced sputum and saliva. Clin Exp Allergy 2005;35(9):1180–5.

74. Lemière C. Non-invasive assessment of airway inflammation in occupational lung diseases. Curr Opin Allergy Clin Immunol 2002;2(2):109–14.

75. Seltzer J, Bigby BG, Jeffery PK, et al. O3 induced change in bronchial reactivity to methacholine and airway inflammation in humans. J Appl Physiol 1986;60: 1321–6.

76. LeVan TD, Koh WP, Lee HP, et al. Vapor, dust, and smoke exposure in relation to adult-onset asthma and chronic respiratory symptoms. The Singapore Chinese Health Study. Am J Epidemiol 2006;163:1118–28.

77. Tarlo SM. Cough: occupational and environmental considerations. ACCP evidence-based clinical practice guidelines. Chest 2006;129:186–96.

78. American Thoracic Society Statement. Occupational contribution to the burden of airway disease. Am J Respir Crit Care Med 2003;167:787–97.

79. Cain WS, Cometto-Muniz JE. Irritation and odor as indicators of indoor pollution. Occup Med 1995;10(1):133–45.

80. Trupin L, Earnest G, Sanpedro M, et al. The occupational burden of chronic obstructive pulmonary disease. Eur Respir J 2003;22:462–9.

81. Tanaka H, Saikai T, Sugawara H, et al. Workplace-related chronic cough on a mushroom farm. Chest 2002;122(3):1080–5.

82. Minnette A. Questionnaire of the European Community for Coal and Steel (ECSC) on respiratory symptoms. 1987—updating of the 1962 and 1967 questionnaires for studying chronic bronchitis and emphysema. Eur J Respir Dis 1989;2:165–77.

83. Groneberg DA, Nowak D, Wussow A, et al. Chronic cough due to occupational factors. J Occup Med Toxicol 2006;1(3):1–10.

84. Gordon SB, Curran AD, Turley A, et al. Glass bottle workers exposed to low-dose irritant fumes cough but do not wheeze. Am J Respir Crit Care Med 1997;156(1):206–10.

85. Gordon SB, Curran AD, Turley A, et al. Respiratory symptoms among glass bottle workers–cough and airways irritancy syndrome? Occup Med (Lond) 1998;48(7):455–9.

86. Blanc PD, Liu C, Juares C, et al. Cough in hot pepper workers. Chest 1991;99: 27–32.
87. Niimi A, Torrego A, Nicholson AG, et al. Nature of airway inflammation and remodeling in chronic cough. J Allergy Clin Immunol 2005;116:565–70.
88. Holgate ST, Davies DE, Lackie PM, et al. Epithelial-mesenchymal interactions in the pathogenesis of asthma. J Allergy Clin Immunol 2000;105(2):193–204.
89. Lemière C, Malo JL, Boutet M. Reactive airways dysfunction syndrome due to chlorine: sequential bronchial biopsies and functional assessment. Eur Respir J 1997;10:241–4.
90. Crystal RG, Randell SH, Engelhardt JF, et al. Airway epithelial cells: current concepts and challenges. Proc Am Thorac Soc 2008;5:772–7.
91. Zhang Y, Goss AM, Cohen ED, et al. A Gata6-Wnt pathway required for epithelial stem cell development and airway regeneration. Nat Genet 2008;40: 862–70.
92. Busse WW, Coffman RL, Gelfand EW, et al. Mechanisms of persistent airway inflammation in asthma. A role for T cells and T-cell products [review]. Am J Respir Crit Care Med 1995;152(1):388–93.
93. Fahy JV, Corry DB, Boushey HA. Airway inflammation and remodeling in asthma [review]. Curr Opin Pulm Med 2000;6(1):15–20.
94. Lee LY, Widdicombe JG. Modulation of airway sensitivity to inhaled irritants: role of inflammatory mediators [review]. Environ Health Perspect 2001;4:585–9.
95. Holgate ST. The airway epithelium is central to the pathogenesis of asthma. Allergol Int 2008;57:1–10.
96. Woolf CJ, Ma Q. Nociceptors—noxious stimulus detectors. Neuron 2007;55: 353–64.
97. Taylor-Clark T, Undem BJ. Transduction mechanisms in airway sensory nerves. J Appl Physiol 2006;101:950–9.
98. Brooks SM. Irritant-induced chronic cough: irritant-induced TRPpathy. Lung 2008;186:S88–93.
99. Brooks SM. Occupational, environmental, and irritant induced cough. Otolaryngol Clin North Am 2010;43:85–96.
100. Nilius B, Voets T, Peters I. TRP channels in disease. Sci STKE 2005;295:1–9.
101. Rohacs T, Nilius B. Regulation of transient receptor potential (TRP) channels by phosphoinositides. Pflugers Arch 2007;455:157–68.
102. Tatar M, Pecova R. The effect of experimental gastroesophageal reflux on the cough reflex in anesthetized cats. Bratisl Lek Listy 1996;97(5):284–8 [in Slovak].
103. Wong CH, Matai R, Morice AH. Cough induced by low pH. Respir Med 1999; 93(1):58–61.
104. Clapham DE. TRP channels as cellular sensors. Nature 2003;426:517–24.
105. Huang CL. The transient receptor potential superfamily of ion channels. J Am Soc Nephrol 2004;15:1690–9.
106. Groneberg DA, Niimi A, Dinh QT, et al. Increased expression of transient receptor potential vanilloid-1 in airway nerves of chronic cough. Am J Respir Crit Care Med 2004;170:1276–80.
107. Groneberg DA, Quarcoo D, Frossard N, et al. Neurogenic mechanisms in bronchial inflammatory diseases. Allergy 2004;59(11):1139–52.
108. Birrell MA, Belvisi MG, Grace M, et al. TRPA1 agonists evoke coughing in guinea pig and human volunteers. Am J Respir Crit Care Med 2009;180:1042–7.
109. Bautista DM, Jordt SE, Nikai T, et al. TRPA1 mediates the inflammatory actions of environmental irritants and proalgesic agents. Cell 2006;124:1269–82.

110. Bautista DM, Movahead P, Hinman A, et al. Pungent products from garlic activate the sensory ion channel TRPA1. Proc Natl Acad Sci U S A 2005;102: 12248–52.
111. Trevisani M, Siemens J, Matwrazzi S, et al. 4-Hydroxynonenal, an endogenous aldehyde, causes pain and neurogenic inflammation through activation of the irritant receptor TRPA1. Proc Natl Acad Sci U S A 2007;104:13519–24.
112. Mcnamara CR, Mandel-Brehm J, Bautista DM, et al. TRPA1 mediates formalin-induced pain. Proc Natl Acad Sci U S A 2007;104:13525–30.
113. Gatti R, Andre E, Amadesi S, et al. Protease-activated receptor-2 exaggerates TRPV1-mediated cough in guinea pigs. J Appl Physiol 2006;101:506–11.
114. Nakatsuka T, Gu JG. P2x purinoceptors and sensory transmission. Pflugers Arch 2006;452:598–607.
115. Vaughan R, Szewczyk JM, Lanos M, et al. Adenosine sensory transduction pathways contribute to activation of the sensory irritation response to inspired irritant vapors. Toxicol Sci 2006;93:411–21.
116. Lee LY, Kwong K, Lin YS, et al. Hypersensitivity of bronchopulmonary C-fibers induced by airway mucosal inflammation: cellular mechanisms. Pulm Pharmacol Ther 2002;15(3):199–204.
117. Choudry NB, Fuller RW, Pride NB. Sensitivity of the human cough reflex: effect of inflammatory mediators prostaglandin E2, bradykinin, and histamine. Am Rev Respir Dis 1989;140(1):137–41.
118. Stone R, Barnes PJ, Fuller RW. Contrasting effects of prostaglandins E2 and F2 alpha on sensitivity of the human cough reflex. J Appl Physiol 1992;73(2): 649–53.
119. Chambers LS, JI B, Ge Q, et al. Par-2 activation, PGE2, and COX-2 in human asthmatic and nonasthmatic airway smooth muscle. Am J Physiol Lung Cell Mol Physiol 2003;285:L619–27.
120. Amadesi S, Nie J, Vergnolle N, et al. Protease-activated receptor-2 sensitizes the capsaicin receptor transient receptor potential vanilloid receptor 1 to induce hyperalgesia. J Neurosci 2004;24:4300–12.
121. Morgan RK, Costello RW, Durcan N, et al. Diverse effects of eosinophil cationic granule proteins on IMR-32 nerve cell signaling and survival. Am J Respir Cell Mol Biol 2005;33:169–77.
122. Lazaar AL, Panettieri J, Reynold A. Airway smooth muscle: a modulator of airway remodeling in asthma. J Allergy Clin Immunol 2005;116(3):488–95.
123. Chung KF, Adcock IM. Pathophysiological mechanisms of asthma. Application of cell and molecular biology techniques. Mol Biotechnol 2001;18(3):213–32.
124. Doherty MJ, Mister R, Pearson MG, et al. Capsaicin responsiveness and cough in asthma and chronic obstructive pulmonary disease. Thorax 2000;55(8): 643–9.
125. Folkerts G, Nijkamp FP. Virus-induced airway hyperresponsiveness. Role of inflammatory cells and mediators [review]. Am J Respir Crit Care Med 1995; 151(5):1666–73.
126. Karlsson JA, Zackrisson C, Lundberg JM. Hyperresponsiveness to tussive stimuli in cigarette smoke-exposed guinea-pigs: a role for capsaicin-sensitive, calcitonin gene-related peptide-containing nerves. Acta Physiol Scand 1991; 141(4):445–54.
127. Olgart C, Frossard N. Nerve growth factor and asthma. Pulm Pharmacol Ther 2002;15(1):51–60.
128. Jacoby DB. Airway neural plasticity. The nerves they are a-changin'. Am J Respir Cell Mol Biol 2003;28:138–41.

129. Quarcoo D, Schulte-Herbruggen O, Lommatzsch M, et al. Nerve growth factor induces increased airway inflammation via a neuropeptide-dependent mechanism in a transgenic animal model of allergic airway inflammation. Clin Exp Allergy 2004;34:1146–51.

130. Karjalainen A, Martikainen R, Karjalainen J, et al. Excess incidence of asthma among Finnish cleaners employed in different industries. Eur Respir J 2002; 19(1):90–5.

131. Medina-Ramon M, Zock JP, Kogevinas M, et al. Asthma symptoms in women employed in domestic cleaning: a community based study. Thorax 2003; 58(11):950–4.

132. Rosenman KD, Reilly MJ, Schill DP, et al. Cleaning products and work-related asthma. J Occup Environ Med 2003;45(5):556–63.

133. Reinisch F, Harrison RJ, Cussler S, et al. Physician reports of work-related asthma in California, 1993-1996. Am J Ind Med 2001;39(1):72–83.

134. Arif AA, Delclos GL, Lee ES, et al. Prevalence and risk factors of asthma and wheezing among US adults: an analysis of the NHANES III data. Eur Respir J 2003;21(5):827–33.

135. Kogevinas M, Anto JM, Sunyer J, et al. Occupational asthma in Europe and other industrialised areas: a population-based study. Lancet 1999;353(9166): 1750–4.

136. Prezant DJ, Weiden M, Banauch GI, et al. Cough and bronchial responsiveness in firefighters at the World Trade Center site. N Engl J Med 2002;347:806–15.

137. Landrigan PJ, Lioy PJ, Thurston G, et al. NIEHS World Trade Center Working Group. Health and environmental consequences of the World Trade Center disaster. Environ Health Perspect 2004;112:731–9.

138. Gavett SH, Haykal-Coates N, Highfill JW, et al. World Trade Center fine particulate matter causes respiratory tract hyperresponsiveness in mice. Environ Health Perspect 2003;111:981–91.

139. Rom WN, Welden M, Garcia R, et al. Acute eosinophilic pneumonia in a New York city firefighter exposed to World Trade Center dust. Am J Respir Crit Care Med 2002;166:797–800.

140. Banauch GI, Alleyne D, Sanchez R, et al. Persistent hyperreactivity and reactive airway dysfunction in firefighters at the World Trade Center. Am J Respir Crit Care Med 2003;168(1):54–62.

141. Hazucha MJ, Bates DV, Bromberg PA. Mechanism of action of ozone on the human lung. J Appl Physiol 1989;67:1535–41.

142. Bates DV, Bell GM, Burnham CD, et al. Short-term effects of ozone on the lung. J Appl Physiol 1972;32:176–81.

143. Hazucha MJ, Folinsbee J, Bromberg PA. Distribution and reproducibility of spirometric response to ozone by gender and age. J Appl Physiol 2003;95: 1917–25.

144. Foster WM, Brown R, Macri K, et al. Bronchial reactivity of healthy subjects: 18-20 h postexposure to ozone. J Appl Physiol 2000;89:1804–10.

145. Holz O, Jorres RA, Timm P, et al. Ozone-induced airway inflammatory changes differ between individuals and are reproducible. Am J Respir Cell Mol Biol 1999; 159:776–84.

146. Coleridge JC, Coleridge HM, Schelegle ES, et al. Acute inhalation of ozone stimulates bronchial C-fibers and rapidly adapting receptors in dogs. J Appl Physiol 1993;74:2345–52.

147. Gavett SH, Kollarik M, Undem BJ. Irritant agonists and air pollutants: neurologically medicated respiratory and cardiovascular responses. In: Foster WM,

Costa DL, editors. Air pollutants and the respiratory tract, vol. 204. 2nd edition. Boca Raton (FL): Taylor And Francis Group; 2005. p. 195–232.

148. Graham RM, Friedman M, Hoyle GW. Sensory nerves promote ozone-induced lung inflammation in mice. Am J Respir Crit Care Med 2001;164:307–11.

149. Basha MJ, Gross KB, Gwizdala CJ, et al. Bronchoalveolar lavage neutrophilia in asthmnatics and healthy volunteers after controlled exposure to ozone and filtered purified air. Chest 1994;106:1757–65.

150. Devlin R, Mcdonnell W, Mann R, et al. Exposure of humans to ambient levels of ozone for 6.6 hours causes cellular and biochemical changes in the lung. Am J Respir Cell Mol Biol 1991;4:72–81.

151. Jorres RA, Holz O, Zachgo W, et al. The effects of repeated ozone exposure on inflammatory markers in bronchoalveolar lavage fluid and mucosal biopsies. Am J Respir Crit Care Med 2000;161:1855–61.

152. Koren HS, Bromberg PA. Respiratory responses of asthmatics to ozone. Int Arch Allergy Immunol 1995;107(1–3):236–8.

153. Kreutzer R, Neutra RR, Lashuay N. Prevalence of people reporting sensitivities to chemicals in a population-based survey. Am J Epidemiol 1999;150:1–17.

154. Baldwin CM, Bell IR, O'rourke MK, et al. The association of respiratory problems in a community sample with self-reported chemical intolerance. Eur J Epidemiol 1997;13:547–52.

155. Bell IR, Schwartz GE, Peterson JM, et al. Self-reported illness from chemical odors in young adults without clinical syndromes or occupational exposures. Arch Environ Health 1993;48:6–13.

156. Ternesten-Hasseus E, Farbrot A, Lowhagen O, et al. Sensitivity to methacholine and capsaicin in patients with unclear respiratory symptoms. Allergy 2002;57: 501–7.

157. Millqvist E. Cough provocation with capsaicin is an objective way to test sensory hyperreactivity in patients with asthma-like symptoms. Allergy 2000; 55:546–50.

158. Ternesten-Hasseus E, Lowhagen O, Millqvist E. Quality of life and capsaicin sensitivity in patients with airway symptoms induced by chemicals and scents: a longitudinal study. Environ Health Perspect 2007;115:425–9.

159. Millqvist E, Lowhagen O, Bende M. Quality of life and capsaicin sensitivity in patients with sensory airway hyperreactivity. Allergy 2000;55:540–5.

160. Kongerud J. Respiratory disorders in aluminum potroom workers. Med Lav 1992;83(5):414–7.

161. Kongerud J, Boe J, Soyseth V, et al. Aluminum potroom asthma: the Norwegian experience. Eur Respir J 1994;7(1):165–72.

162. Soyseth V, Kongerud J, Ekstrand J, et al. Relation between exposure to fluoride and bronchial responsiveness in aluminum potroom workers with work-related asthma-like symptoms. Thorax 1994;49(10):984–9.

163. Desjardins A, Bergeron JP, Ghezzo H, et al. Aluminum potroom asthma confirmed by monitoring of forced expiratory volume in one second. Am J Respir Crit Care Med 1994;150(6 Pt 1):1714–7.

164. Pavord ID, Brightling CE, Woltmann G, et al. Non-eosinophilic corticosteroid unresponsive asthma. Lancet 1999;353(9171):2213–4.

165. Brightling CE. Chronic cough due to nonasthmatic eosinophilic bronchitis. ACCP evidence-based clinical practice guidelines. Chest 2006;129(Suppl 1): 116s–21s.

166. Gibson PG, Dolovich J, Denburg J, et al. Chronic cough: eosinophilic bronchitis without asthma. Lancet 1989;1:1346–8.

167. Quirce S. Eosinophilic bronchitis in the workplace. Curr Opin Allergy Clin Immunol 2004;4(2):87–91.

168. Perkner JJ, Fennelly KP, Balkissoon R, et al. Irritant-associated vocal cord dysfunction. J Occup Environ Med 1998;40(2):136–43.

169. Huggins JT, Kaplan A, Martin-Harris B, et al. Eucalyptus as a specific irritant causing vocal cord dysfunction. Ann Allergy Asthma Immunol 2004;93(3): 299–303.

170. Tarlo SM. Workplace respiratory irritants and asthma. Occup Med 2000;15(2): 471–84.

171. Sokol WN, Aelony Y, Beall GN. Meat wrapper's asthma: an appraisal of a new occupational syndrome. J Allergy Clin Immunol 1973;226:448–54.

172. Brooks SM, Vandervort R. Polyvinyl chloride film thermal decomposition products as an occupational illness of meat wrappers: II clinical studies. J Occup Med 1977;19:192–6.

173. Karpati AM, Perrin MC, Matte T, et al. Pesticide spraying for West Nile virus control and emergency department asthma visits in New York city, 2000. Environ Health Perspect 2004;112(11):1183–7.

174. Salameh PR, Baldi I, Brochard P, et al. Respiratory symptoms in children and exposure to pesticides. Eur Respir J 2003;22(3):507–12.

175. Cone JE, Wugofski L, Balmes Jr, et al. Persistent respiratory health effects after metam sodium pesticide spill. Chest 1994;106:500–8.

176. Brooks SM, Spaul W, McCluskey JD. The spectrum of building-related airway disorders: difficulty in retrospectively diagnosing building-related asthma. Chest 2005;128:1720–7.

177. Rumchev KB, Spickett JT, Bulsara MK, et al. Domestic exposure to formaldehyde significantly increases the risk of asthma in young children. Eur Respir J 2002;20(2):403–8.

178. Hendrick DJ, Rando RJ, Lane DJ, et al. Formaldehyde asthma: challenge exposure levels and fate after five years. J Occup Med 1982;24(11):893–7.

179. Pratt PC, Vollmer RT, Miller JA. Epidemiology of pulmonary lesions in nontextile and cotton textile workers. Chest 1980;35:133–8.

180. Richards I, Kulkarni A, Brooks SM, et al. Florida red-tide toxins (brevotoxins) produce depolarization of airway smooth muscle. Toxicon 1990;28:1105–11.

181. Savonius B, Keskinen H, Tuppurainen M, et al. Occupational asthma caused by ethanolamines. Allergy 1994;49(10):877–81.

182. Goh CL. Common industrial processes and occupational irritants and allergens—an update. Ann Acad Med Singapore 1994;23(5):690–8.

183. Boswell RT, Mccunney RJ. Bronchiolitis obliterans from exposure to incinerator fly ash. J Occup Environ Med 1995;37:850–5.

184. Markopoulo KD, Cool CD, Elliott TL, et al. Obliterative bronchiolitis: varying presentations and clinicopathological correlation. Eur Respir J 2002;19: 20–30.

185. Myers J, Colby T. Pathological manifestations of bronchiolitis, constrictive bronchiolitis, cryptogenic organizing pneumonia, and diffuse panbronchiolitis. Clin Chest Med 1993;14:611–22.

186. Ryu JH, Myers JL, Swenson SJ. Bronchiolar disorders. Am J Respir Crit Care Med 2003;168:1277–92.

187. Schacter EN. Popcorn worker's lung (editorial). N Engl J Med 2002;347:360–1.

188. Parmet AJ, Von Essen S. Rapidly progressive, fixed airway obstructive disease in popcorn workers: a new occupational pulmonary illness? J Occup Environ Med 2002;44:216–8.

189. Akpinar-Elci M, Travis WD, Lynch DA, et al. Bronchiolitis obliterans syndrome in popcorn production plant workers. Eur Respir J 2004;24:298–302.
190. Hubbs AF, Battelli L, Goldsmith WT, et al. Necrosis of nasal and airway epithelium in rats inhaling vapors of artificial butter flavoring. Toxicol Appl Pharmacol 2002;185:128–35.
191. Kreiss K, Gomaa A, Kullman G, et al. Clinical bronchiolitis obliterans in workers at a microwave-popcorn plant. N Engl J Med 2002;347:330–8.

Hypersensitivity Pneumonitis and Related Conditions in the Work Environment

Michael C. Zacharisen, MD*, Jordan N. Fink, MD

KEYWORDS

- Hypersensitivity pneumonitis • Extrinsic allergic alveolitis
- Occupational

Hypersensitivity pneumonitis, also known as extrinsic allergic alveolitis, is an uncommon non–immunoglobulin E (IgE), T-helper cell type 1 (Th1)–mediated inflammatory pulmonary disease with systemic symptoms resulting from repeated inhalation and subsequent sensitization to a large variety of aerosolized antigenic organic dust particles. The exaggerated immune response to repeated inhalation of these particles leads to infiltration and proliferation of activated pulmonary macrophages and lymphocytes, resulting in lymphocytic alveolitis and bronchiolitis with noncaseating granulomas. Fibrosis may occur with chronic exposure. Recurrent or chronic cough and/or dyspnea with or without systemic symptoms should alert the physician to the diagnosis. The earliest forms of hypersensitivity pneumonitis were related to farming and, each year, new antigens causing occupational disease are described.

Hypersensitivity pneumonitis was originally described in 1713 as an occupational lung disease in grain workers and later, in 1932, in farmers inhaling moldy hay contaminated with thermophilic actinomyces, hence the term farmer's lung.[1] With this recognition, modernization of farming methods has resulted in the reduction in farmer's lung prevalence estimated at 0.5% to 3% of exposed farmers in studies spanning from 1980 to 2003. Definite conclusions on prevalence and incidence of farmers lung are elusive because of methodological issues in study design and definitions of disease, fewer farmers in general, and erroneous diagnoses.[2] However, farming continues to represent a major source of exposure to antigens capable of causing occupational

Funding support: None.
The authors have nothing to disclose.
Department of Pediatrics, Medical College of Wisconsin, 9000 West Wisconsin Avenue, Suite 411, Milwaukee, WI 53226, USA
* Corresponding author.
E-mail address: mzachari@mcw.edu

Immunol Allergy Clin N Am 31 (2011) 769–786
doi:10.1016/j.iac.2011.07.004
0889-8561/11/$ – see front matter © 2011 Elsevier Inc. All rights reserved.

immunology.theclinics.com

hypersensitivity pneumonitis. National surveillance screening in the United Kingdom from 1992 to 2001 estimated 50 cases of hypersensitivity pneumonitis annually, representing 1.8% of all cases of work-related respiratory disease seen by chest physicians. For occupational physicians, the average annual rate of hypersensitivity pneumonitis was 1 per million employees, representing about 4 cases per year or 0.7% of all work-related respiratory disease.[3]

SPECIFIC OCCUPATIONS AND WORK-RELATED ANTIGENS

Many diverse occupations in which workers are exposed to antigens small enough to reach the distal airway (<5 μm) have been implicated as inducing hypersensitivity pneumonitis (**Table 1**). These antigens include organic dusts containing bacteria, fungi,[4] animal or plant proteins, or low-molecular-weight chemicals.

Farming

Farmer's lung is the prototype occupational hypersensitivity pneumonitis. The antigens of farmer's lung vary between countries and within countries depending on the climate and the methods of farming and hay production used. Many forms of farmer's lung are now fungal induced and include a worker sorting onions and potatoes[5]; workers in large and small commercial indoor mushroom farms[6]; and workers exposed to moldy crops of grapes, tobacco,[7] sugarcane,[8] and peat moss.[9] Agricultural exposures were the most common occupation for hypersensitivity pneumonitis in the Czech Republic, with 69% of cases of farmer's lung (cattleman and dairyman), followed by malt workers and chemical workers.[10] A report of coffee-worker's lung was reconsidered after a patient developed additional laboratory and clinical findings consistent with cryptogenic fibrosing alveolitis associated with rheumatoid arthritis.[11]

Animal and Bird Raising Industry

A quality control worker in a feed factory developed acute disease after taking samples of cattle feed treated with phytase, a fungal-derived enzyme used to treat cattle feed to strengthen bone.[12] Historically, feather bloom and droppings from pigeons or indoor pet birds have been implicated in triggering pigeon breeder's lung or bird fancier's disease. Occupations with bird antigen exposure include keeping domesticated fowl (chicken, turkey) and game farms raising pheasants.[13]

Machinists

More than a dozen outbreaks of hypersensitivity pneumonitis affecting hundreds of workers exposed to contaminated airborne synthetic metalworking fluids (MWF) have been reported since the mid-1990s.[14] This disorder is presumed to be related to the increased use of water-based fluids and automation of high-speed machining processes resulting in the generation of airborne aerosols. MWF are used during grinding, drilling, cutting, and shaping metal to cool, lubricate, and remove metal particles thus prolonging the life of the machinery. Although MWFs contain biocides, they are prone to contamination of rapidly growing *Mycobacterium immunogenum* and *Pseudomonas* species that form biofilms that line the pipes, pumps, and containers and are resistant to treatment.[15] The current Occupational Safety and Health Administration (OSHA) standard for allowable oil mist exposure of 5 mg/m^3 does not prevent hypersensitivity pneumonitis. Despite multiple publications on the health effects of MWF, legal action from union groups, and recommendations from the National Institute for Occupational Safety and Health (NIOSH) to lower the exposure limit to 0.5 mg/m^3, no further action has been taken and court challenges have been denied.[16]

Table 1
Antigens of occupational hypersensitivity pneumonitis

Occupation	Source	Antigen	Disease
Farming	Hay/silage	Thermophilic actinomycetes *Saccharopolyspora rectivirgula* *Lichtheimia corymbifera* (France) *Eurotia amstelodami* *Wallemia sebi* (Finland)	Farmer's lung
	Grain[a]	*Aspergillus fumigatus*	
	Moldy sugar cane	*Thermoactinomyces sacchari*	Bagassosis
	Tobacco	*Aspergillus*	Tobacco workers' disease
	Moldy grapes	*Botrytis cinerea*	Wine grower's lung
	Peat moss	*Penicillium* sp, *Monocillium*	Peat moss processor's lung
	Moldy onions or potatoes	*Fusarium, Penicillium* sp	
	Mushrooms	*Penicillium citrinum*	Mushroom picker's lung
Animal/bird industry	Cattle feed	Phytase enzyme[a]	
	Veterinary feed	Soybean hulls	
	Feather bloom, droppings	Pheasant	Pheasant rearer's lung
Food Industry			
Sausage/salami makers	Dry sausage molds	*Penicillium camembertii*	
Cheese makers	Moldy cheese	*Penicillium roqueforti*	Cheese worker's lung
Mill workers	Wheat flour (contaminated)	*Sitophilus* (wheat weevil)	Wheat weevil disease
Malt workers	Moldy brewing malt[a]		Malt worker's lung
Soy sauce brewer	Soy sauce production	*Aspergillus oryzae*	
Laboratory workers	Laboratory reagent	Pauli reagent	Pauli HP
	Rodents[a]	Rat or gerbil urinary proteins	Gerbil keeper's lung
Textile/clothing industry	Nylon plant air-conditioning	*Cytophaga* producing endotoxin	
	Silk production	Silkworm larvae cocoon fluff	Sericulturist's lung disease
	Hair and fur from pelts	Proteins in animal fur dust[a]	Furrier's lung
	Button making	Mollusk/oyster shell dust	
Machine operators	Metal working fluids[a]	*Mycobacterium immunogenum, Pseudomonas*	Machine operator's lung
Detergent industry	Enzyme dust[a]	*Bacillus subtilis*	Enzyme worker's lung

(continued on next page)

Table 1 (continued)			
Occupation	Source	Antigen	Disease
Professional musician	Trombone	*Mycobacterium chelonae* or *Fusarium*	Trombone player's lung
Medical/dental	Dental prosthesis production	Methylmethacrylate	
Stucco workers	Plaster for stucco	Thermophilic or *Aspergillus*	Stipatosis
Polyurethane industry	Foam production	Isocyanates[a]	
	Yacht making	Dimethylphthalate or styrene	Yacht-maker's lung
	Epoxy resin	Phthalic anhydrides	
Wood processing plants	Wood dust	Cabreuva, pine sawdust	Wood worker's lung
	Moldy wood planks	*Paecilomyces*	Woodman's disease
	Cork dust	Cork proteins or mold (*Penicillium glabrum*)	Suberosis
	Moldy maple bark	*Cryptosroma corticale*	Maple bark strippers disease
	Moldy wood dust	*Alternaria, Rhizopus, Mucor*	Wood trimmer's disease
	Moldy redwood dust	*Pullaria*	Sequoiosis

[a] Antigens also implicated in occupational asthma.

The number of new cases of MWF-induced hypersensitivity pneumonitis is difficult to determine because of the sporadic nature of the outbreaks and the possibility of underreporting. The last major outbreak, published in 2007, reported on 19 workers diagnosed between 2003 and 2004 in a car engine manufacturing plant in the United Kingdom.[17] The number of published reports on outbreaks has decreased from 4 in 2003 to 1 report annually from 2005 to 2007 and none in the last 3 years.

Food Industry

Food-related occupations have been associated with fungus-induced occupational hypersensitivity pneumonitis in cheese (blue and Gruyere),[18] malt,[19,20] and sausage[21] workers and even in a soy sauce brewer.[22]

Textile/Clothing Industry

Workers developed disease after sawing nacre (mother-of-pearl) used to make buttons.[23] The inhalation of hair and dust by furriers working with fox and other pelts led to disease with hair shafts found in the granulomas on lung biopsy.[24] In the process of collecting silk for making garments, inhalational exposure to the cocoon fluff containing larval proteins can trigger disease termed sericulturist's lung.[25]

Industrial Exposures of Low-Molecular-Weight Chemicals

Workers exposed to isocyanates during the production of polyurethane foam, elastomers, adhesives, and paints have developed hypersensitivity pneumonitis. In 2008, a secretary in a car body repair shop exposed to low amounts of diisocyanates developed the subacute form.[26] Phthalates or styrene was implicated in a woman rolling panels in making yacht hulls[27] or phthalic anhydrides in epoxy resin workers.[28]

Woodworkers

Either wood itself or fungal-contaminated wood can induce hypersensitivity pneumonitis in sensitized workers. Mold-contaminated wood dust has been reported to cause hypersensitivity pneumonitis in tree trimmers, sawmill workers, lumberjacks, and wood pulp workers.[29] A worker installing parquet floors made of cabreuva wood developed acute disease caused by the wood dust itself.[30] Cork dust containing suberin cork protein and fungal-colonized cork (*Penicillium*, *Aspergillus*, *Mucor*, *Rhizopus*) led to hypersensitivity pneumonitis in cork workers termed suberosis and first identified in 1955.[31]

Rare Causes

Case reports of hypersensitivity pneumonitis have included a worker that inhaled 1,1,1,2-tetrafluoroethane (HFC134a) coolant as part of laser hair removal.[32] In Spain, stucco workers were exposed to either esparto grass (*Stipa tenacissima*) termed stipatosis or to grass contaminated with thermophilic actinomycetes or *Aspergillus*.[33] Workers using enzymes may develop occupational asthma or hypersensitivity pneumonitis from *Bacillus subtilis* exposure.[34]

IMMUNOPATHOPHYSIOLOGY

The pathogenesis of hypersensitivity pneumonitis is complex and still not fully understood.[35] The duration and degree of antigen exposure necessary to sensitize and induce symptoms is also not known.

Although many workers are exposed to potentially sensitizing organic dusts, few develop hypersensitivity pneumonitis, which suggests a genetic susceptibility. Genetic susceptibility is associated with polymorphisms in (1) the promoter region in the tumor necrosis factor (TNF)-α gene on chromosome 6[36]; (2) the low-molecular-weight proteosome genes that affect the enzymatic function of protein degradation into peptides for presentation in the major histocompatibility complex (MHC) class 1 pathway[37]; and (3) in transporters associated with antigen processing (TAP) genes for MHC class I molecules.[38]

Environmental factors associated with an increased risk of developing disease include high insecticide exposures[39] and influenza viral infections.[40] Nicotine in cigarette smoke affects alveolar function, thus downregulating the inflammatory effect, resulting in less-acute hypersensitivity pneumonitis in smokers but a worse prognosis for those who develop the chronic form. Other factors that may contribute to hypersensitivity pneumonitis are abnormal surfactant and low levels of antioxidant enzymes in alveoli.[41]

A Th1 immune response with Gell and Coombs type III immune complex and type IV cell-mediated mechanisms seems to be involved. After inhalation of small organic antigens into the alveoli, alveolar macrophages become activated and release Th1-associated inflammatory cytokines including TNF-α, interleukin (IL)-1, IL-8, and IL-12. The antigen can have direct nonspecific actions including complement activation via the alternate pathway leading to vascular permeability related to C3a and chemoattraction of neutrophils and macrophages via C5a. The antigen can also interact with toll-like receptor 2 (TLR2) and MyD88 for neutrophil recruitment.[42] After interaction with CD8+ T cells, IL-2, IL-8, IL-12, IL-16, IL-18, and interferon γ (IFN-γ) are released and IL-10 is reduced.[43] IFN-γ is responsible for granuloma formation. Chemokines such as IL-8 in the acute phase attract neutrophils into the airway that release potent mediators such as hydroxyl anions and toxic oxygen species. An influx of CD8+ lymphocytes and eosinophils releasing inflammatory factors promotes airway inflammation, activates endothelium, and leads to collagen synthesis by secreting glycoproteins capable of leading to airways fibrosis. T regulatory cells in patients with hypersensitivity pneumonitis are nonfunctional and unable to suppress the uncontrolled inflammation, possibly through increased IL-17 production.[44] Decreased lymphocyte apoptosis leads to airways lymphocytosis possibly through antiapoptotic cytokines.

In mouse models, the enhanced maturation of antigen-presenting CD11c+ cells explains the virus-induced enhanced immune response to farmer's lung antigens.[45] The overexpression of GATA binding protein 3 transcription factor, which participates in Th2 differentiation, attenuates the development of hypersensitivity pneumonitis by correcting the Th1-polarizing condition.[46] Mice models may not simulate human disease in all cases.

CLASSIFICATIONS

Despite the wide variety of antigens responsible, the clinical features of hypersensitivity pneumonitis are essentially the same with recurrent respiratory and systemic features or insidious respiratory and systemic symptoms depending on frequency and intensity of exposure of the organic dust. There is overlap of the various forms. Traditionally, the classifications have been clinically divided into acute, subacute, and chronic forms.[47] Other approaches suggested are to view the disease as active versus sequelae or as recurrent systemic with normal chest radiographs versus those with features of advanced interstitial disease on high-resolution computed tomography (HRCT), resting hypoxemia, and a restrictive pattern on lung function.[48]

Acute Form

In a sensitized worker, within 4 to 6 hours (up to 22 hours) of significant antigen exposure, flulike symptoms with high fever, chills, sweating, body aches, nonproductive cough, chest tightness, dyspnea, and malaise occur, with spontaneous resolution within 24 hours of avoidance of the inciting antigen. Subsequent antigen exposures result in similar symptoms with variable intensity depending on the antigen load. Recurrent acute episodes may lead to chronic symptoms and lung function changes even after antigen exposure ceases.

Subacute Form

In the sensitized worker, repeated low-level antigen exposures during weeks to months can result in an indolent and subtle presentation with progressive cough and dyspnea on exertion. Although high fever is lacking, nonspecific systemic symptoms of anorexia and malaise may occur. This classification is more difficult to define.

Chronic Form

The chronic form is subdivided into chronic insidious and chronic recurrent. Continuous low-level exposure results in a slowly progressive course with insidious exertional dyspnea during months to years with anorexia, weight loss, weakness, and fatigue. In contrast, recurrent acute episodes can progress to chronic disease.

DIAGNOSIS

Like other occupational disorders, the clinician must first confirm the diagnosis of hypersensitivity pneumonitis and then identify the relationship to workplace exposures. At the current time, there is no single diagnostic study or biomarker to confirm hypersensitivity pneumonitis. Instead, an assemblage of signs, symptoms, and laboratory, radiologic, and lung function studies can support the diagnosis (**Box 1**).[49] To assess for an antigen that is of occupational origin, a detailed, targeted, and extended occupational history is required. Frequently, a team approach including industrial hygienist, allergist, pulmonologist, and occupational physician is necessary. A sentinel case should prompt additional inquiries into the worksite processes and exposures and seek to identify other exposed workers with disease.

History and Physical Examination

A detailed history of symptoms and exposures is critical to determining the correct diagnosis. Work history should include details on current and previous occupations with attention to work processes and exposures to chemicals, dusts, and aerosols. This history should include use of personal respiratory protective equipment, work-place ventilation, shifts worked, and whether symptoms occur away from work. Review of material safety data sheets and a personal worksite assessment may be necessary. The collection of dust, fumes, and water/fluid samples for staining and culture may assist in identifying the causative antigen. Information on maintenance records and sick days can be reviewed. Improvement of symptoms away from work and/or a rapid response to oral steroids should heighten the awareness of occupational hypersensitivity pneumonitis.

The physical examination can be completely normal between acute episodes. With acute symptoms, the worker appears extremely ill, tachypneic and dyspneic without rhinitis, pharyngitis, or conjunctivitis. Lung auscultation reveals fine, bibasilar, end-inspiratory rales and, occasionally, diffuse wheezing. Rash, adenopathy, cardiac, joint, and abdominal symptoms are absent. In the chronic form, the worker may appear well at rest, but may be dyspneic with minor activity, show clubbing of the digits, and exhibit rales or wheezing on lung auscultation.

Box 1
Occupational hypersensitivity pneumonitis: diagnosis

Major Criteria (requires at least 2):

1. Symptoms compatible with hypersensitivity pneumonitis

2. Exposure to an antigen by history or detection of antibody in serum or bronchoalveolar lavage (BAL) fluid

3. Chest radiograph or HRCT with compatible findings

4. Lymphocytosis in lung lavage fluid if BAL is performed

5. Compatible histopathologic changes on lung biopsy, if biopsy is performed

6. Reproduction of symptoms and laboratory and lung function abnormalities after exposure to the suspect workplace

Minor Criteria:

1. Dyspnea on exertion

2. Bibasilar dry inspiratory crackles

3. Recurrent febrile episodes

4. Decreased lung diffusion capacity (DLCO)

5. Arterial hypoxemia at rest or with exercise

Pulmonary Function Testing

Spirometry, lung volumes, and diffusing capacity should be obtained to assess impairment and guide therapy. Between attacks, pulmonary function may be normal. In acute disease, a restrictive pattern with declines in forced vital capacity (FVC) and forced expiratory volume in 1 second (FEV_1) is usually observed with normal peak expiratory flows within 6 hours of antigen exposure. The diffusing capacity as measured by DLCO is reduced, consistent with impaired alveolar function. Arterial blood gas measurement reveals hypoxemia with exercise and, in some cases, at rest. A biphasic response with reductions in FVC and FEV_1 1 to 2 hours after antigen exposure, and again 4 to 6 hours after exposure, has been described. In the chronic form, workers may have a mixture of restrictive and obstructive lung disease patterns with an inconsistent response to bronchodilator. Methacholine challenge tests are frequently normal but, in chronic disease, can be positive. Exhaled nitric oxide was increased in 1 case.[50]

Chest Radiography

Findings suggestive of acute hypersensitivity pneumonitis include bilateral diffuse ground-glass infiltrate, patchy opacifications in lower lung fields, and interstitial infiltrates or a fine nodular or reticulonodular pattern (**Fig. 1**). These findings are completely reversible. Up to 30% of patients may have a normal radiograph. In the subacute form, fine nodular opacities reflecting granulomas may be observed. The chronic form is characterized by reticular opacities, fibrosis, honeycombing, and volume loss.[51] Notably absent are single nodular lesions, hilar adenopathy, consolidations, and pleural effusions.

Thin-section computed tomography (CT) or HRCT using 0.5-mm to 1-mm slice thickness provides a highly detailed image that is fundamental in identifying and quantifying severity in diffuse parenchymal and interstitial lung diseases as well as identifying coexisting or alternative diagnoses.[52] In acute/subacute disease, ground-glass attenuation is seen in the bilateral middle lung zones and fine, centrilobular micronodules are found primarily in the midlung to lower lung zones. In the chronic forms, irregular linear opacities, volume loss, traction bronchiectasis, and honeycombing suggest fibrosis. Other findings include emphysema and mosaic patterns from combinations of

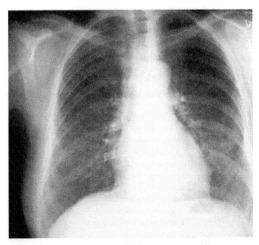

Fig. 1. Chest radiograph of acute hypersensitivity pneumonitis.

ground-glass attenuation and air trapping.[53] Mediastinal adenopathy less than 20 mm in diameter are seen with HRCT in more than 25% of cases.

Laboratory Studies

Symptomatic workers with the acute form typically have leukocytosis with a left shift and occasionally eosinophilia up to 20%. Serum complement, erythrocyte sedimentation rate (ESR), C-reactive protein (CR-P), and lactate dehydrogenase (LDH) may be increased, but are not necessarily useful in monitoring disease activity. Quantitative serum immunoglobulins (Ig; IgA, IgG, IgM) may be increased, except IgE. Although antinuclear antibodies are negative, rheumatoid factor (RF) may be positive. Serum precipitating antibody to antigen as identified by Ouchterlony gel technique or other IgG immunoassays is the classic immunologic finding confirming exposure to the putative offending antigen. (**Fig. 2**) Serum precipitins may wane with time if antigen exposure ends. Up to 50% of similarly exposed asymptomatic workers may have detectable antibodies without apparent disease. Negative commercial antibody panels in a confirmed clinical case may result from using incorrect antigens, low serum concentrations of antibody, or from nonstandardized antigens. Newer serologic techniques such as electrosyneresis on cellulose acetate may be more discriminating for patients compared with healthy exposed workers.[54] In vitro lymphocyte transformation studies using specific antigen are positive in symptomatic patients but also in up to 15% of asymptomatic, similarly exposed individuals. Skin-prick testing is unnecessary because the pathogenesis is not IgE mediated and intradermal skin testing can result in both false-positive and false-negative reactions.

BAL

BAL can assist in excluding other interstitial lung disorders and reveal consistent findings in cell types.[55] In nonexposed, asymptomatic individuals, low numbers of CD4+ lymphocytes and alveolar macrophages predominate. The results are dependent on the timing of the last antigen exposure. Neutrophils are increased within 48 hours

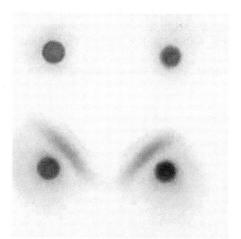

Fig. 2. Serum precipitins as shown by the Ouchterlony double immunodiffusion gel system. The intensity of the stained bands between the central well (barely visible) containing antigen and the 2 lower wells containing patient serum indicates the presence of precipitating antigen-antibody complexes. The upper 2 wells contain serum that does not have antibody against the antigen being tested.

and return to normal levels within 1 week. In symptomatic or exposed and nonsymptomatic nonsmoking workers, BAL reveals high numbers (>50% lymphocytes) of both CD4+ and CD8+ lymphocytes. These levels may remain increased for years and wane in time if further antigen exposure is avoided. Current smokers may have lower percentages of alveolar lymphocytes. The symptomatic worker with acute disease who is a nonsmoker, exhibits a predominately CD8+ response resulting in a low CD4+/CD8+ ratio whereas a worker with the chronic/fibrotic form or in those who smoke is likely to have a predominance of CD4+ T cells thus increasing the CD4+/CD8+ ratio. Compared with other interstitial lung diseases, there are increased mast cells and plasma cells. A normal BAL excludes hypersensitivity pneumonitis.[56] In nonsmokers, BAL lymphocytes less than 30% make the diagnosis unlikely. Pulmonary sarcoidosis classically presents with a predominance of CD4+ T cells and high CD4+/CD8+ ratio. Cultures are typically negative.

Histopathology

Although a tissue diagnosis is not required, it may eliminate other diseases in the differential diagnosis. Video-assisted thoracoscopic surgery (VATS) for biopsy is becoming the procedure of choice for lung biopsy because of its lower morbidity and mortality, shorter hospital stay, and good diagnostic yield.[57] Transbronchial biopsies may not obtain adequate samples for representative pathology. The classic triad of findings is lymphoplasmocytic interstitial infiltrate, poorly formed nonnecrotizing granulomas, and cellular bronchiolitis (**Fig. 3**). Depending on the stage of disease and intensity of antigen exposure, the findings may range from the acute form with neutrophils, activated foamy macrophages, prominent lymphocytic alveolitis, plasma cells, and granulomas in up to 70% compared with the subacute and chronic forms having a nonspecific interstitial pneumonia (NSIP) pattern or usual interstitial pneumonia (UIP) pattern without granulomas.[58,59] A difficult problem is prognosis and therapeutic decisions for the patient with irrefutable idiopathic pulmonary fibrosis IPF/UIP with relevant antigen exposure and positive serum precipitins . Antigen avoidance and corticosteroid therapy may occasionally delay or prevent progression of fibrotic hypersensitivity pneumonitis. Similarly, if the CT scan shows findings of fibrotic end-stage UIP, the value of a biopsy should be weighed against the risks of the procedure. Even in the chronic form, with a UIP-like pattern, centrilobular and bridging fibrosis are important hallmarks of chronic hypersensitivity pneumonitis with less than half showing granulomas. These patterns can also be seen in connective tissue disorders

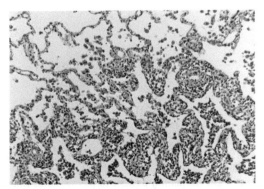

Fig. 3. Low-power view of a lung biopsy revealing noncaseating granulomas and lymphocytic interstitial infiltrate.

and pneumotoxic drug reactions.[60] Recently, a subgroup of patients have been identified that have both hypersensitivity pneumonitis and a rare condition termed pulmonary alveolar proteinosis. The link between these distinct disorders is unclear.[61] Vasculitis and connective tissue destruction should prompt an evaluation for other causes.

Inhalation Challenge

A natural challenge at the workplace after a period of avoidance can precipitate symptoms and show laboratory and lung function changes, but not necessarily confirm the specific causative antigen. A purposeful challenge to a suspect antigen using a nebulizer is typically reserved for unique cases or clinical research when a new antigen is being investigated. Because of a lack of standardized antigens (imprecise mixtures of antigen and nonspecific irritants) and techniques and the risk of significant symptoms, the challenge should be performed by qualified personnel in specialized centers with experience. A positive challenge is represented by cough and dyspnea, increased body temperature, peripheral leukocytosis, and decrements in FVC and oxygen saturation usually occurring 4 to 6 hours after exposure. As an example, in Montreal, Canada, in 2009, an inhalation challenge was performed for malt dust. Lactose inhaled by a particle generator was used as the control with FVC and FEV_1 measurements. For the next 2 days, aerosolized malt dust via a particle generator was administered for 30 minutes with similar spirometric measurements and oral temperatures. Methacholine challenge was performed after the second day of malt dust inhalation. The next day, 120 minutes of malt dust exposure were followed by serial spirometric measurements at 10, 40, 60, 90, 120, 180, 240, 300, 360, and 420 minutes as well as serial oral temperature measurements. After symptoms occurred, diffusion capacity, blood gas measurement for oxygen tension, chest radiograph, and blood counts for leukocytes and neutrophils were obtained.[20] The diagnosis of malt-induced hypersensitivity pneumonitis was confirmed.

DIFFERENTIAL DIAGNOSIS

Many disorders may mimic occupational hypersensitivity pneumonitis and should be considered in the evaluation of individual workers (**Table 2**).

Berylliosis

Although acute berylliosis resembling a chemical pneumonitis is rare, chronic beryllium disease (CBD) or berylliosis from exposure in industries such as nuclear reactors and weapons, aerospace, ceramics, dental supplies, and others results in a granulomatous lung response identical to sarcoidosis.[62] The lymphocyte transformation test that quantifies the proliferation of lymphocytes incubated with beryllium is always positive in patients with CBD if BAL lymphocytes are used, but in only 50% of cases if peripheral blood cells are used.[63] Findings on CT not seen in hypersensitivity pneumonitis include hilar or mediastinal lymph nodes with amorphous or eggshell calcification.

Endotoxin-induced Disease

Monday morning fever refers to flulike symptoms that occur on the first day of the work week without radiologic abnormalities or long-term changes in lung function and is likely caused by inhalation of endotoxin. Humidifier fever refers to contaminated humidification or cooling equipment used during a manufacturing process. The gram-negative bacteria *Cytophaga* was identified in a nylon plant, leading to workers

Table 2
Differential diagnosis of occupational hypersensitivity pneumonitis

Acute Form	Disorder	Trigger
Farming	Silo unloader's disease	Nitrogen dioxide
Organic dust toxic syndrome	Humidifier fever, animal house fever, grain fever, pulmonary mycotoxicosis	Endotoxin, mycotoxin
Inorganic dust toxic syndrome	Acute berylliosis	Beryllium dust: aerospace, nuclear, ceramics, dental
Textile dust	Byssinosis Mill fever Weaver's cough	Cotton dust and endotoxin Tannins in cotton mill dust, kapok Tamarind seed powder
Bird raising	Psittacosis	*Chlamydia psittaci* infection
Chronic Form		
Inorganic respiratory dust syndromes	Silicosis and siderosis	Silica in mining, quarrying, drilling, foundry working, ceramics manufacturing, sandblasting
	Chronic berylliosis	Beryllium dust -aerospace, nuclear, ceramics, dental
	Asbestosis	Fibrous silicate minerals (eg, chrysotile)
	Coal worker's pneumoconiosis	Mixed dust consisting of coal, kaolin, mica
	Talcosis and calcicosis	Leather, ceramic, paper, plastics, rubber, building, paint, or cosmetic industries; limestone dust
Food industry	Flavor-worker's lung	Diacetyl butter flavor ketone in microwave popcorn
	Rice-miller's syndrome	Rice husk dust containing silica
Textile dust	Byssinosis Nylon flock Ardystil syndrome	Cotton, hemp, flax, jute, sisal Pulverized fibers applied to fabrics Acramin-FWN (a polyamidoamine)
Lifeguards	Lifeguard lung	Trichloramine and/or endotoxin
Office buildings	Sick building syndrome	VOC, smoke, poor ventilation, dampness

Abbreviation: VOC, volatile organic compound.

with symptoms.[64] Lung function is either normal or shows mild airway obstruction with normal DLCO. Lifeguard lung is a condition of workers at indoor swimming pools contaminated with gram-negative bacteria and high levels of endotoxin. Although features include lymphocytic alveolitis and noncaseating granulomas, as seen in hypersensitivity pneumonitis, the high attack rate after a short duration of exposure suggests a toxic response.[65] Alternatively, when the disinfectant chlorine combines with nitrogen-containing compounds like sweat and urine, indoor airborne concentrations of trichloramine can increase in pool water to levels causing eye and lung irritation.[66] The levels correlate with the number of occupants in the pool.

Diacetyl Flavoring–induced Bronchiolitis Obliterans

In 2000, workers in microwave popcorn plants exposed to diacetyl flavorings experienced rapid progression to obliterative bronchiolitis and severe airway obstruction without reversibility.[67,68] Clinical findings include chronic nonproductive cough, wheezing, and progressive dyspnea.

Siderosis and Silicosis

Inhalation of fine iron particles by welders using electric arc or oxyacetylene may result in the accumulation of iron oxide in pulmonary macrophages leading to siderosis. Functional impairment and fibrosis are uncommon and the radiological abnormalities resolve with avoidance. In the iron ore mining and processing industry, if silica is involved, silicosiderosis can develop. Silicosis may develop after a latency period of 10 to 30 years after inhaling silica dust during work in mining, quarrying, drilling, foundry work, ceramics manufacturing, and sandblasting. Multiple small nodules are often seen on HRCT in both disorders.

Talcosis and Calcicosis

Hydrated magnesium silicate, known as talc, may be inhaled during processing in the leather, ceramic, paper, plastics, rubber, building, paint, or cosmetic industries, leading to nonnecrotizing pulmonary inflammation. Recreational intravenous drug use has been associated with talcosis. Inhaling limestone dust containing calcium carbonate, magnesium oxide, silica dioxide, and aluminum oxide may result in calcicosis. Widespread nodules are seen on HRCT and histology reveals numerous birefringent crystals consistent with limestone.

Ardystil Syndrome

Inhalation of Acramin-FWN (polyamidoamine) by employees in the textile industry during its application with a brush or sponge for printing resulted in organizing pneumonia.[69] Progressive interstitial fibrosis could evolve into respiratory failure with a poor prognosis.

Organic Dust Toxic Syndrome

Farmers may develop cough and chest tightness after exposure to inhaling dense clouds of dust when working with swine, poultry, or grains. Multiple workers are usually affected. Fungal spores and increases of total cells are found in BAL. The exact trigger is unclear, but may include endotoxin, ammonia, and/or hydrogen sulfide gases. Symptoms resolve quickly and spontaneously with complete recovery. In a population-based survey, California farmers exposed to agricultural dust self-reported a high incidence of persistent wheeze and other respiratory symptoms, asthma, and bronchitis.[70] Personal respiratory protection was rarely used. Malaysian workers inhaling rice husk dust during milling developed acute and chronic irritant effects of the eyes and skin, rhinitis, asthma, eosinophilia, or interstitial lung disease without restriction, postulated to be related to deposition of the elongated spikes on the rice husks shown on electron microscopy.[71]

Sick Building Syndrome

The working population spends about 20% of its time at work. Since the 1970s, in buildings designed and manufactured for maximum efficiency, groups of workers have presented with nonspecific complaints affecting their eyes, skin, and upper airways, as well as headache and fatigue without objective findings, radiologic abnormalities, or lung function changes. Several factors associated with sick building syndrome (SBS) include relative air humidity, temperature, building dampness, air ventilation, tobacco smoke, chemical indoor exposures (volatile organic compounds, ozone, formaldehyde), and video display terminal work. Workers with certain personality characteristics such as anxiety, depression, and neuroticism are more likely to experience SBS. Furthermore, a psychosocial work environment where workers have high demands but lack control and lack support from superiors and colleagues was more common in SBS.[72]

TREATMENT
Avoidance

As with other occupational lung diseases, the obvious and most important treatment is avoidance of the triggering antigen. Frequently, this is sufficient intervention and can be accomplished by removing and replacing the antigen with a nonsensitizing alternative, altering the process to prevent antigen from becoming airborne, or moving the worker away from the exposure. On occasion, the specific antigen is elusive despite establishing the worksite as causative. Wearing well-fitted, appropriate respiratory protection with filters can be effective when complete avoidance is not possible.

Examples of successful avoidance measures for MWF include changes in engineering such as enclosing machines, improving ventilation, and wearing personal respiratory protection as well as treatment and replacement of metalworking fluids to decrease the bacterial contamination. Effective concentrations of biocides containing methyloxazolidine can reduce the growth and proliferation of *Mycobacterium* species in water-based machining coolants. Simple dipslides can monitor the effectiveness of this approach.[73]

For farmer's lung, changes in storing process or treating hay with buffered propionic acid significantly reduced the concentration of thermophilic bacteria and fungi without affecting the machinery or cattle. Job retraining and changing professions are usually reserved for when avoidance measures are insufficient because this extracts a financial and emotional toll on both workers and employers.

Pharmacologic Therapy

In acutely ill workers with abnormal lung function and chest radiograph changes, supplemental oxygen and parenteral corticosteroids are recommended. Prednisone at 40 to 80 mg daily for 1 to 2 weeks may be sufficient for acute disease, whereas a gradual taper lasting weeks to months may be necessary for those with subacute or chronic disease, depending on their response to treatment. Case reports have shown improvement with inhaled beclomethasone 400 μg daily in hydrofluoroalkane propellant or inhaled budesonide after either oral or pulse intravenous infusions of corticosteroids, respectively. If reversible airway obstruction is shown, short-acting β bronchodilators and inhaled corticosteroids can be used. In vitro studies have shown promise for thalidomide, pentoxifylline, low-dose, long-term macrolide antibiotics, and cyclosporine, but controlled clinical trials have not been performed.

PROGNOSIS

For acute or subacute disease, early recognition and treatment results in complete recovery unless permanent damage has occurred. Unrecognized hypersensitivity pneumonitis with ongoing antigen exposure may result in permanent sequelae. The clinical course is variable, as shown by progression of symptoms despite avoidance measures in some individuals, whereas other workers remain stable despite continued exposure. Fibrosis, as seen in the chronic form or a UIP-like pattern, portends a generally poor prognosis with median survival of 2 years compared with 22 years in the subacute form in which no fibrosis is present.[58] Oral steroids may improve symptoms, but have not been shown to affect the long-term prognosis. Although tobacco smokers are less likely to develop acute hypersensitivity pneumonitis, they may experience a worse outcome from progression of the chronic form.

SUMMARY OF IMPORTANT POINTS

Hypersensitivity pneumonitis can occur from a wide variety of occupational exposures in which workers inhale fungi, bacteria, animal emanations, or low-molecular-weight chemicals. Although uncommon and difficult to recognize, through a detailed work exposure history, physical examination, radiography, pulmonary function studies, and selected laboratory studies using sera and BAL fluid, workers can be identified early to effect avoidance of the antigen and institute pharmacologic therapy if necessary. A lung biopsy may be necessary to rule out other interstitial lung diseases. Despite the varied organic antigen triggers, the presentation is similar with acute, subacute, or chronic forms. Systemic corticosteroids are the only reliable pharmacologic treatment but do not alter the long-term outcome.

REFERENCES

1. Pepys J, Jenkins PA, Festenstein GN, et al. Farmer's lung: thermoactinomyces as a source of farmer's lung antigen. Lancet 1963;2:607–11.
2. Lacasse Y, Cormier Y. Hypersensitivity pneumonitis. Orphanet J Rare Dis 2006;1:25.
3. McDonald JC, Chen Y, Zekveld C, et al. Incidence by occupation and industry of acute work related respiratory diseases in the UK, 1992–2001. Occup Environ Med 2005;62:836–42.
4. Selman M, Lacasse Y, Pardo A, et al. Hypersensitivity pneumonitis caused by fungi. Proc Am Thorac Soc 2010;7:229–36.
5. Merget R, Sander I, Rozynek P, et al. Occupational hypersensitivity pneumonitis due to molds in an onion and potato sorter. Am J Ind Med 2008;51:117–9.
6. Tanaka H, Sugawara H, Saikai T, et al. Mushroom worker's lung caused by spores of *Hypsizigus marmoreus* (Bunashimeji): elevated serum surfactant protein D levels. Chest 2000;118:1506–9.
7. Huuskonen M, Husman K, Jarvisalo J, et al. Extrinsic allergic alveolitis in the tobacco industry. Br J Ind Med 1984;41:77–83.
8. Romeo L, Dalle Molle K, Zanoni G, et al. Respiratory health effects and immunological response to *Thermoactinomyces* among sugar cane workers in Nicaragua. Int J Occup Environ Health 2009;15:249–54.
9. Cormier Y, Israël-Assayag E, Bédard G, et al. Hypersensitivity pneumonitis in peat moss processing plant workers. Am J Respir Crit Care Med 1998;158:412–7.
10. Fenclova Z, Pelclova D, Urban P, et al. Occupational hypersensitivity pneumonitis reported to the Czech national registry of occupational diseases in the period 1992–2005. Ind Health 2009;47:443–8.
11. Van den Bosch J, Van Toorn D, Wagenaar S. Coffee-worker's lung: reconsideration of a case report. Thorax 1983;38:720.
12. van Heemst RC, Sander I, Rooyackers J, et al. Hypersensitivity pneumonitis caused by occupational exposure to phytase. Eur Respir J 2009;33:1507–9.
13. Partridge S, Pepperell J, Forrester-Wood C, et al. Pheasant rearer's lung. Occup Med 2004;54:500–3.
14. Bernstein DI, Lummus ZL, Santilli G, et al. Machine operator's lung: a hypersensitivity pneumonitis disorder associated with exposure to metalworking fluids aerosols. Chest 1995;1008:636–41.
15. Rosenman KD. Asthma, hypersensitivity pneumonitis and other respiratory diseases caused by metalworking fluids. Curr Opin Allergy Clin Immunol 2009;9:97–102.

16. Mirer FE. New evidence on the health hazards and control of metalworking fluids since completion of the OSHA advisory committee report. Am J Ind Med 2010;53: 792–801.

17. Robertson W, Robertson AS, Burge CB, et al. Clinical investigation of an outbreak of alveolitis and asthma in a car engine manufacturing plant. Thorax 2007;62: 981–90.

18. Campbell J, Kryda J, Treuhaft MW, et al. Cheese workers' hypersensitivity pneumonitis. Am Rev Respir Dis 1983;127:495–6.

19. Blyth W, Grant W, Blackadder E, et al. Fungal antigens as a source of sensitization and respiratory disease in Scottish maltworkers. Clin Allergy 1977;7:549–62.

20. Miedinger D, Malo JL, Cartier A, et al. Malt can cause both occupational asthma and allergic alveolitis. Allergy 2009;64:1228–9.

21. Rouzaud P, Soulat J, Trela C, et al. Symptoms and serum precipitins in workers exposed to dry sausage mould: consequences of exposure to sausage mould. Int Arch Occup Environ Health 2001;74:371–4.

22. Tsuchiya Y, Shimokata K, Ohara H, et al. Hypersensitivity pneumonitis in a soy sauce brewer caused by *Aspergillus oryzae*. J Allergy Clin Immunol 1993;91: 688–9.

23. Orriols R, Aliaga J, Antó JM, et al. High prevalence of mollusc shell hypersensitivity pneumonitis in nacre factory workers. Eur Respir J 1997;10:780–6.

24. Pimentel J. Furrier's lung. Thorax 1970;25:387–98.

25. Nakazawa T, Umegae Y. Sericulturist's lung disease: hypersensitivity pneumonitis related to silk production. Thorax 1990;45:233–4.

26. Schreiber J, Knolle J, Sennekamp J, et al. Sub-acute occupational hypersensitivity pneumonitis due to low-level exposure to diisocyanates in a secretary. Eur Respir J 2008;32:807–11.

27. Volkman K, Merrick J, Zacharisen M. Yacht-maker's lung: a case of hypersensitivity pneumonitis in yacht manufacturing. WMJ 2006;105:47–50.

28. Piirilä P, Keskinen H, Anttila S, et al. Allergic alveolitis following exposure to epoxy polyester powder paint containing low amounts(<1%) of acid anhydrides. Eur Respir J 1997;10:948–51.

29. Dykewicz M, Laufer P, Patterson R, et al. Woodman's disease: hypersensitivity pneumonitis from cutting live trees. J Allergy Clin Immunol 1988;81:455–60.

30. Baur X, Gahnz G, Chen Z. Extrinsic allergic alveolitis caused by cabreuva wood dust. J Allergy Clin Immunol 2000;106:780–1.

31. Morell F, Roger A, Cruz M, et al. Suberosis: clinical study and etiologic agents in a series of 8 patients. Chest 2003;124:1145–52.

32. Ishiguro T, Yasui M, Nakade Y, et al. Extrinsic allergic alveolitis with eosinophil infiltration induced by 1,1,1,2-tetrafluoroethane (HFC-134a): a case report. Intern Med 2007;46:1455–7.

33. Moreno-Ancillo A, Dominguez-Noche C, Carmen Gil-Adrados A, et al. Familial presentation of occupational hypersensitivity pneumonitis caused by *Aspergillus*-contaminated esparto dust. Allergol Immunopathol (Madr) 2003;31: 294–6.

34. Tripathi A, Grammer L. Extrinsic allergic alveolitis from a proteolytic enzyme. Ann Allergy Asthma Immunol 2001;86:425–7.

35. Girard M, Israel-Assayag E, Cormier Y, et al. Pathogenesis of hypersensitivity pneumonitis. Curr Opin Allergy Clin Immunol 2004;4:93–8.

36. Camarena A, Juarez A, Mejia M, et al. Major histocompatibility complex and tumor necrosis factor-alpha polymorphisms in pigeon breeder's disease. Am J Respir Crit Care Med 2001;163:1528–33.

37. Camarena A, Aquino-Galvez A, Falfan-Valencia R, et al. PSMB8 (LMP7) but not PSMB9 (LMP2) gene polymorphisms are associated to pigeon breeder's hypersensitivity pneumonitis. Respir Med 2010;104:889–94.
38. Aquino-Galvez A, Camarena A, Montano M, et al. Transporter associated with antigen processing (TAP) 1 gene polymorphisms in patients with hypersensitivity pneumonitis. Exp Mol Pathol 2008;84:173–7.
39. Hoppin J, Umbach D, Kullman G, et al. Pesticides and other agricultural factors associated with self-reported farmer's lung among farm residents in the Agricultural Health Study. Occup Environ Med 2007;64:334–41.
40. Dakhama A, Hegele R, Laflamme G, et al. Common respiratory viruses in lower airways of patients with acute hypersensitivity pneumonitis. Am J Respir Crit Care Med 1999;159:1316–22.
41. Behr J, Degenkolb B, Beinert T, et al. Pulmonary glutathione levels in acute episodes of farmer's lung. Am J Respir Crit Care Med 2000;161:1968–71.
42. Nance S, Yi A, Re F, et al. MyD88 is necessary for neutrophil recruitment in hypersensitivity pneumonitis. J Leukoc Biol 2008;83:1207–17.
43. Ye Q, Nakamura S, Sarria R. Interleukin 12, interleukin 18, and tumor necrosis factor release by alveolar macrophages: acute and chronic hypersensitivity pneumonitis. Ann Allergy Asthma Immunol 2009;102:149–54.
44. Girard M, Israel-Assayag E, Cormier Y. Impaired function of regulatory T cells in hypersensitivity pneumonitis. Eur Respir J 2011;37(3):632–9.
45. Girard M, Israel-Assayag E, Cormier Y. Mature CD11c+ cells are enhanced in hypersensitivity pneumonitis. Eur Respir J 2009;34:749–56.
46. Matsuno Y, Ishii Y, Yoh K, et al. Overexpression of GATA-3 protects against the development of hypersensitivity pneumonitis. Am J Respir Crit Care Med 2007;176:1015–25.
47. Richerson HB, Bernstein IL, Fink JN, et al. Guidelines for the clinical evaluation of hypersensitivity pneumonitis: report of the subcommittee on hypersensitivity pneumonitis. J Allergy Clin Immunol 1989;84:839–44.
48. Lacasse Y, Selman M, Costabel U, et al. Classification of hypersensitivity pneumonitis. Int Arch Allergy Immunol 2009;149:161–6.
49. Fink JN, Ortega HG, Reynolds HY, et al. NHLBI workshop: needs and opportunities for research in hypersensitivity pneumonitis. Am J Respir Crit Care Med 2005;171:792–8.
50. Shirai T, Ikeda M, Morita S, et al. Elevated alveolar nitric oxide concentration after environmental challenge in hypersensitivity pneumonitis. Respirology 2010;15:721–5.
51. Hirschmann J, Pipavath S, Godwin J. Hypersensitivity pneumonitis: a historical, clinical, and radiologic review. Radiographics 2009;29:1921–38.
52. Lucía Flors L, Domingo ML, Leiva-Salinas C, et al. Uncommon occupational lung diseases: high-resolution CT findings. AJR Am J Roentgenol 2010;194:20–6.
53. Verschakelen J. The role of high-resolution computed tomography in the work-up of interstitial lung disease. Curr Opin Pulm Med 2010;16:503–10.
54. Reboux G, Piarroux R, Roussel S, et al. Assessment of four serological techniques in the immunological diagnosis of farmer's lung disease. J Med Microbiol 2007;56:1317–21.
55. Reynolds H. Present status of bronchoalveolar lavage in interstitial lung disease. Curr Opin Pulm Med 2009;15:479–85.
56. Cordeiro CR, Jones JC, Alfaro T, et al. Bronchoalveolar lavage in occupational lung diseases. Semin Respir Crit Care Med 2007;28:504–13.

57. Chang AC, Yee J, Orringer MB, et al. Diagnostic thoracoscopic lung biopsy: an outpatient experience. Ann Thorac Surg 2002;74:1942–6.
58. Churg A, Sin DD, Everett D, et al. Pathologic patterns and survival in chronic hypersensitivity pneumonitis. Am J Surg Pathol 2009;33:1765–70.
59. Takemura T, Akashi T, Ohtani Y, et al. Pathology of hypersensitivity pneumonitis. Curr Opin Pulm Med 2008;14:440–54.
60. Antin-Ozerkis D, Rubinowitz A. Update on nonspecific interstitial pneumonia. Clin Pulm Med 2010;17:122–8.
61. Verma H, Nicholson A, Kerr K, et al. Alveolar proteinosis with hypersensitivity pneumonitis: a new clinical phenotype. Respirology 2010;15:1197–202.
62. Maier L. Clinical approach to chronic beryllium disease and other nonpneumoconiotic interstitial lung diseases. J Thorac Imaging 2002;17:273–84.
63. Rossman MD, Kern JA, Elias JA, et al. Proliferative response of bronchoalveolar lymphocytes to beryllium. Ann Intern Med 1988;108:687–93.
64. Nordness M, Zacharisen M, Schlueter D, et al. Occupational lung disease related to *Cytophaga* endotoxin exposure in a nylon plant. J Occup Environ Med 2003; 45:385–92.
65. Rose CS, Martyny JW, Newman LS, et al. "Lifeguard lung": endemic granulomatous pneumonitis in an indoor swimming pool. Am J Public Health 1998;88: 1795–800.
66. Dang B, Chen L, Mueller C, et al. Ocular and respiratory symptoms among lifeguards at a hotel indoor waterpark resort. J Occup Environ Med 2010;52:207–13.
67. Kreiss K, Gomaa A, Kullman G, et al. Clinical bronchiolitis obliterans in workers at a microwave-popcorn plant. N Engl J Med 2002;347:330–8.
68. Kanwal R. Bronchiolitis obliterans in workers exposed to flavoring chemicals. Curr Opin Pulm Med 2008;14:141–6.
69. Sole A, Cordero P, Morales P, et al. Epidemic outbreak of interstitial lung disease in aerographics textile workers - the "Ardystil syndrome": a first year follow up. Thorax 1996;51:94–5.
70. Schenker MB, Farrar JA, Mitchell DC, et al. Agricultural dust exposure and respiratory symptoms among California farm operators. J Occup Environ Med 2005; 47:1157–66.
71. Lim H, Domala Z, Joginder S, et al. Rice millers' syndrome: a preliminary report. Br J Ind Med 1984;41:445–9.
72. Norback D. An update on sick building syndrome. Curr Opin Allergy Clin Immunol 2009;9:55–9.
73. Steinhauer K, Goroncy-Bermes P. Treatment of water-based metalworking fluids to prevent hypersensitivity pneumonitis associated with *Mycobacterium* spp. J Appl Microbiol 2008;104:454–64.

Occupational Rhinitis

J. Wesley Sublett, MD, MPH, David I. Bernstein, MD*

KEYWORDS

- Work-related rhinitis • Work-exacerbated rhinitis
- Occupational rhinoconjunctivitis • Pharmacotherapy
- Immunotherapy

Work-related rhinitis (WRR) is an important occupational disorder that may be more prevalent than work-related asthma (WRA). The prevalence rates of WRR vary widely dependent on the workplace and agent involved. Occupational rhinoconjunctivitis (OR) has been estimated to affect 2% to 87% of workers exposed to occupational allergens and chemical agents.[1]

WRR describes a variety of conditions where nasal symptoms can be triggered from exposure to high molecular weight (HMW) protein allergens, chemical sensitizers, or irritants encountered in the work environment.[2] WRR can be further classified into OR and work-exacerbated rhinitis (WER) (**Fig. 1**). OR can be defined as rhinitis directly attributable to a specific substance or condition encountered in the work environment. Chemical fumes or accidental exposure to high levels of irritants in the workplace can induce chronic rhinitis, which was been termed reactive upper airways dysfunction syndrome (RUDS). Consistent with the aforementioned definition, this syndrome would be considered a nonallergic form of OR.

OR should be distinguished from WER, or a pre-existing rhinitis condition (eg, allergic rhinitis) worsened by circumstances (eg, irritants contained in environmental tobacco smoke) encountered in the work environment. That is, WER is not induced or caused by workplace exposures. Due to the limited published evidence related to WER, this article will concentrate on the discussion of mechanisms, epidemiology, diagnosis, and management of OR.

MECHANISMS

Both allergic and nonallergic mechanisms can be involved in OR. OR is commonly associated with allergic sensitization to HMW protein allergens. Rarely, low molecular weight (LMW) chemical sensitizers can form allergens by haptenizing with respiratory proteins and elicit typical allergic rhinoconjunctivitis symptoms at work.

Allergic OR is best characterized by nasal and ocular symptoms due to an agent that has induced immunoglobulin E (IgE)-mediated sensitization. Development of allergic

Division of Immunology, Allergy and Rheumatology, University of Cincinnati College of Medicine, 3255 Eden Avenue, Cincinnati, OH 45267-0563, USA
* Corresponding author.
E-mail address: david.i.bernstein@uc.edu

Immunol Allergy Clin N Am 31 (2011) 787–796
doi:10.1016/j.iac.2011.07.007
0889-8561/11/$ – see front matter © 2011 Elsevier Inc. All rights reserved.

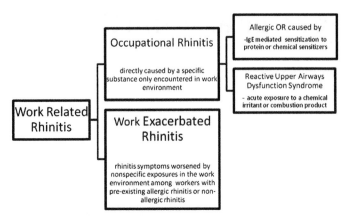

Fig. 1. Classification of work-related rhinitis.

OR symptoms is preceded by a latency period of exposure of months to years. Occupational allergens are derived from either animal or plant proteins. Demonstration of allergic sensitization is necessary to confirm allergic OR by a positive skin prick test or elevated serum-specific IgE to the suspect workplace allergen(s). A few reactive chemicals, such as the acid anhydrides (phthalic anhydride, trimellitic anhydride) and platinum salts, have the capacity to haptenize, forming allergenic epitopes known to elicit specific IgE responses. After a latency period of exposure to these chemicals during which IgE-mediated sensitization occurs, affected workers develop OR and OA symptoms.[3,4] To confirm sensitization to acid anhydrides, skin prick testing or serum-specific IgE immunoassays can be performed with antigens prepared by conjugating chemical (eg, trimellitic anhydride) with human serum albumin.

RUDS, a phenotype of nonallergic OR, is chronic rhinitis related to an acute exposure to a chemical irritant or combustion products. Onset of this condition is not preceded by a latency period. Nasal pathology in RUDS is characterized by focal epithelial desquamation, glandular hypertrophy, lymphocytic infiltrates, and sensory nerve fiber proliferation. Substance P released from sensory nerves, and not histamine, is hypothesized as the major mediator involved.[5]

EPIDEMIOLOGY AND WORK EXPOSURES INVOLVED IN OR

OR may occur in a diverse number of occupational settings. As mentioned, causes are typically categorized into HMW and LMW compounds. HMW exposures are usually proteins of biologic origin. LMW compounds are chemicals that can act as an irritants sometimes inducing RUDS or triggering WER, or rarely act as sensitizers.[1,2,6]

Prevalence rates for OR associated with HMW compounds have varied from 2% to 87%. Lower prevalence rates (3%–48%) are reported with OR caused by exposure to LMW compounds.[1]

SPECIFIC CAUSATIVE AGENTS

Although many occupational environments present risks for development of OR, few of these have been well characterized. **Table 1** summarizes well-described occupations associated with OR. Studies involving laboratory animal workers exposed to exposed to rats, mice, rabbits, guinea pigs, hamsters, dogs, cats, and monkeys report a prevalence ranging from 10% to 33%; OR was 2 to 4 times more common than OA in

Table 1
Agents and occupations in work-related rhinitis

Agent	Occupation
Low Molecular Weight Agents	
Anhydrides	Chemical workers
	Epoxy resin production workers
Diisocyanates	Carpenters
	Furniture makers
	Painters
	Urethane mold workers
Drugs	Health care workers
	Pharmaceutical workers
Metals	Platinum refinery workers
Wood dust	Carpenters
	Furniture makers
Other chemicals	Cobblers
	Hairdressers
	Paper mill workers
	Reactive dye production workers
	Textile workers
High Molecular Weight Agents	
Animal allergens	Laboratory workers
	Swine confinement workers
	Textile workers
	Veterinarians
Biologic Enzymes	Bakers
	Detergent Industry workers
	Pharmaceutical workers
Fish and seafood proteins	Aquarists
	Fish food factory workers
	Seafood packing and processing
Grain and flour dust	Bakers
	Flour packers
	Grain elevator workers
Insects and mites	Bakers
	Farm workers
	Janitorial workers
	Laboratory workers
Latex	Glove manufacturing workers
	Health care workers
	Textile factory workers
Plant allergens	Coffee workers
	Farm workers
	Lawn maintenance workers
	Tobacco manufacturing workers

affected laboratory animal workers.[1] The mean period of latent exposure before onset of OR symptoms in animal workers is 2.3 years, but can range widely from 1 to 18 years.[7] Animal allergens implicated in OR include rats, mice, rabbits, guinea pigs, dogs, foxes, minks, pigs, raccoons, and hens.[7] Animal workers with laboratory animal allergy, especially those exposed to rodents, are at risk for OR.[1,7–13] Reported sensitization to animal allergens, confirmed by skin prick testing or specific IgE antibodies, is 6% to 46% of exposed laboratory animal workers.[1,7–9,12] WER is possible among laboratory animal workers, as studies report 33% to 51% of exposed workers with workplace rhinitis symptoms were sensitized to rat, mice, or guinea pig.[7,8]

The prevalence of OR among bakers is 18% to 29%, compared with 4.9% to 10% of bakers estimated to have OA (ie, bakers' asthma).[1,14–17] Allergen sources are found in flour, including cereal proteins (rye, wheat, barley), grain mites, flour beetles, *Aspergillus fumigatus*, and microbial enzymes (α-amylase, glucoamylase, cellulase).[14–17] Other flour allergens that have been purified and well characterized include: barley glycerinaldehyde-3-phosphate dehydrogenases, barley triosephosphate isomerase, ceral serpins, wheat, and maize thioredoxins.[18,19] OR symptoms begin a mean duration of 11.6 months after initiation of work.[15] Sensitization to flour allergens develops in 10% and 38% of bakers.[1] It appears that 1.7% to 5.2% of bakers are presensitized to bran flour, oatmeal flour, rye flour, and wheat flour before being hired,[14,15] increasing the likelihood of developing WRR by sixfold compared with nonsensitized workers.[14]

OR occurs in health care workers, especially those exposed to natural rubber latex (NRL) and psyllium.[1,20–22] Psyllium, a major component of powdered bulk-forming laxatives, has been reported to cause OR in 9% to 32% of health care workers exposed to psyllium powder.[1] The prevalence of OR ranges from 9% to 34% in NRL sensitized health care workers exposed to gloves and other medical products that contain NRL.[1,20] The mean latency period of exposure before onset of OR symptoms was 5.2 years in NRL-sensitized health care workers.[20] Prior to the reduction of *Hevea brasiliensis* protein allergens in NRL glove products, 5% to 10% of health care workers were skin prick test NRL sensitized.[1] For the past decade, the rates of sensitization and clinical allergy have dramatically decreased due to the introduction of non-NRL substitutes and low-allergen NRL gloves.[23]

Biologic microbial enzymes are used as ingredients in detergents, animal feed, fuel alcohol, textile, paper products, and pharmaceuticals. These are produced by bioengineered *Aspergillus* fungi or bacterial (*Bacillus subtilis*) species. These are extremely potent sensitizers even at low ambient concentrations that can induce allergic rhinitis and OA in large proportions of exposed workers.[1,24–26] In a large, retrospective cohort study, 3% of sensitized workers reported rhinoconjunctivitis symptoms in workers exposed to multiple microbial enzymes (proteases, lipases, cellulases, carboxyhydrases).[24] Similarly, 2 cross-sectional studies have noted that 4.6% to 19% of workers sensitized to microbial enzymes reported upper respiratory symptoms.[25,26]

Diisocyanates, used worldwide in the manufacturing of rigid and flexible polyurethane foam, elastomers, adhesives, paints and varnishes, textiles, and insecticides, are a common cause of OA as well as OR. Few studies have examined the association of diisocyanates with upper airway symptoms. Cross-sectional studies, examining various diisocyanates (hexamethylene diisocyanate, methylene diphenyl diisocyanate, toluene diisocyanate), report 17% to 92% of exposed workers have WRR symptoms.[27–31] However, it remains uncertain as to whether affected workers were experiencing OR or merely work-exacerbated irritant symptoms.

RISK FACTORS ASSOCIATED WITH OR

Exposure level, length of exposure, atopy, and smoking are risk factors associated with the development of OR. The risk of IgE-mediated sensitization to HMW agents is directly related to the level and duration of exposure in workers exposed to laboratory animals,[8,11,12] detergent enzymes,[25,26] flour,[15–17] and α-amylase.[16] Workers exposed to higher levels of HMW agents for extended periods are at greater risk of sensitization and OR symptoms. A cross-sectional study of detergent manufacturing workers demonstrated a significant increase in work-related nasal itch (prevalence ratio [PR], 4.2; 95% confidence interval [CI], 1.5–12), sneezing (PR, 4; 95% CI, 1.5–10.8), and elevated enzyme serum-specific IgE (PR, 3.8; 95% CI, 1–14.1) in those workers who handled enzyme products during the entire work shift compared with workers with incidental exposure.[25] Cross-sectional studies of bakers also demonstrate the prevalence of work-related symptoms and specific IgE antibodies to wheat flour antigens are directly associated with flour dust concentrations.[16,17] A large, prospective study of apprentice bakers further supports that work-related symptoms and sensitization to occupational allergens (bakers' dust, wheat flour, corn flour, rye flour, oatmeal flour, barley flour, threshings) increases with the duration of work exposure as the incidence of reported rhinitis and chest symptoms was 6.5% and 4.2% after 1 year, and 10.8% and 8.6% after 2 years, respectively. This study also reported skin prick sensitization to occupational allergens was found to be 4.6% after 1 year and 8.2% after 2 years.[15]

Atopy, defined by skin prick test positivity to common environmental allergens, is reported to be associated with a greater risk of sensitization to HMW occupational allergens (eg, flour dust, laboratory animals, latex proteins).[1,7,9,14,20] In a prospective study of bakers, workers with positive skin prick test reactivity to grass pollen, cat, or dog allergens confirmed before entry into the work environment were 2 to 3 times more likely to report work-related rhinoconjunctivitis symptoms than nonsensitized workers.[14]

The risk of OR and sensitization to occupational substances association with smoking is unclear. A review examining smoking as a possible risk factor for allergic-sensitization and development of allergic airway diseases concluded that active smoking may enhance risk of sensitization to antigens in flour dust, green coffee beans, castor beans, ispaghula, rat, mouse, guinea pig, rabbit, shellfish, and detergent enzymes.[32] However, subsequent similar studies failed to demonstrate this association.[1,32,33]

RELATIONSHIP BETWEEN OR AND ASTHMA

OA and OR are closely associated and often coexist. The prevalence of OR among workers with confirmed OA is 76% to 92%.[1,34] In a review of OR etiologies, OR was reported to occur 2 to 3 times more frequently than occupational asthma.[1] In a Finnish registry survey of workers reporting OR, 11.6% were confirmed to subsequently develop OA. This study reported a crude incidence rate of asthma of 19 cases per 1000 population per year, and a crude relative risk of asthma of 4.8 (95% CI, 4.3–5.4) for those with OR.[35] OR symptoms typically precede those of OA in 58% of workers exposed to HMW agents and in 25% of workers exposed to LMW agents.[34]

DIAGNOSIS

A diagnosis of OR can be established by a consistent medical history of WRR with or without ocular symptoms combined with demonstration of allergic sensitization to specific substance(s) encountered at work. Nasal congestion, rhinorrhea, and sneezing with nasal, eye, and palatal itching exacerbated by the work environment and resolving on weekends or during vacations are highly consistent with allergic OR. Patients presenting with rhinitis symptoms at work should be evaluated for nonwork-related allergic rhinitis caused by common environmental allergens, which may be confused with OR but more consistent with nonspecific WER. An accurate diagnosis of OR and the ability to distinguish it from WER have important medicolegal consequences, as workers' disability claims are not compensable in many states with a diagnosis of WER or other pre-existing rhinitis conditions.

A specific causative agent can be difficult to identify in complex work environments with exposures to multiple substances. Workers should describe their jobs and industrial processes located in their work area and in adjacent areas. An itemized questionnaire can supplement the physician's interview and prevent omission of important details by capturing essential exposure data and key work-related symptoms.[36,37] Substances to which the patient has direct or indirect exposure should be recorded along with details pertaining to duration and nature of exposure. Physicians can request material safety data sheets to identify exposure to hazardous substances, respiratory irritants, and potential sensitizers.[38] Clinicians should also inquire about accidental chemical spills or fires preceding the development of chronic rhinitis symptoms and perhaps leading to irritant-induced rhinitis (RUDS).

The nasal examination should be performed to exclude nasal polyps or anatomic conditions such as nasal septal deviation. Nasal eosinophils can be identified by scraping or via swab collection from the inferior nasal turbinate, and they can be quantitated. Eosinophils can signify an allergic inflammatory rhinitis due to occupational allergens. However, this finding is not specific for OR, and it can also be present in patients with nonwork-related nonallergic rhinitis with eosinophilia (NARES) or nasal polyposis.[39]

Skin prick testing is preferred, as it is sensitive, rapid, and inexpensive. The lack of commercially available standardized testing extracts for most HMW occupational allergens is a major limitation. If commercially available, US Food and Drug Administration (FDA)-approved serum-specific IgE assays can be quite useful for confirming sensitization, although these are often less sensitive than skin prick testing with standardized skin test allergens (eg, natural rubber latex Hev b allergens).[20]

Acoustic rhinometry uses sound impulse reflections to define the area and dimensions of the upper airways and to help assess nasal patency. It has been demonstrated to correlate well with computed tomography (CT) or magnetic resonance imaging (MRI).[40] The utility of acoustic rhinometry is debatable. In a cross-sectional study of workers exposed to soft paper dust, no difference in intranasal geometry measured by acoustic rhinometry during active exposure in the work environment was reported by workers with nasal obstruction compared with those without nasal obstruction.[41]

Nasal provocation testing (NPT) can confirm specific causative allergens when uncertainty exists regarding the diagnosis or etiology.[40–42] NPT allows direct observation of the causal relationship between exposure to a specific agent and elicitation of rhinitis symptoms. An NPT can be performed in the clinical setting if the agent of interest is available, or it can be performed at the workplace. If the NPT is performed at the workplace, it may not be possible to identify a causative agent due to concomitant exposure to multiple substances in the work environment. Very few specialized centers exist that are equipped to perform clinical NPT with occupational agents.

MANAGEMENT

The first approach in managing WRR is implementation measures to reduce or eliminate exposure to the agent causing the disease. Studies have shown that strategies to reduce occupational exposure have successfully decreased OR symptoms in cases caused by NRL[23] and proteolytic enzymes.[43] Steps to modify the workplace could include: providing adequate ventilation and aspiration of pollutants, using less hazardous materials, and creating closed-circuit manufacturing processes. Workers can be supplied with personal protective equipment, although this strategy is limited by either poor compliance or inability to wear during the long work shift. Respirators are partially effective in reducing symptoms of OR and asthma due to laboratory animals,[10] hexahydrophthalic anhydride (HHPA),[44] and NRL.[45] Subjects with OR are a greater risk for developing OA and should be followed closely to ensure if they remain in the work environment. Those workers who develop OA or rarely anaphylaxis to a workplace allergen must be accommodated, and measures to implement complete avoidance must be instituted.[46]

Pharmacologic therapy for allergic OR is similar to what is used for nonoccupational allergic rhinitis. Nasal steroids are considered first-line therapy for patients with persistent allergic rhinitis. Antihistamines are used for intermittent symptoms or ancillary agents to nasal steroids. Sedating antihistamines should be avoided, particularly if work involves heavy machinery so as to prevent occupational injuries. Sedation and risk are reduced with use of second-generation nonsedating antihistamines.[47]

Allergen immunotherapy (AIT) can be considered in patients with OR caused by allergens for which there are commercially available treatment extracts, in patients who fail to respond to optimal pharmacotherapy, and when causative allergens cannot be avoided. In double-blind placebo-controlled studies, AIT has demonstrated efficacy in treating patients with seasonal and perennial allergic rhinitis caused by pollens and house dust mites.[48] Although studies of AIT's effectiveness in treating OR are lacking, several studies have demonstrated improvement in respiratory symptoms associated with OA.[49] In a study of bakery workers with asthma and wheat flour sensitization, a significant decrease in bronchial hyper-responsiveness and improvement in wheat flour-associated symptoms was seen in workers treated with wheat flour extract AIT.[50] Due to the limited availability of commercial treatment allergens for many forms of allergic OR, indications for AIT are limited to very few occupational allergens. Although similar studies have not been conducted in workers with allergic OR, this is an intriguing possibility that should be addressed in future studies.

SUMMARY

WRR is an important occupational disorder that can affect a diversity of workers and work environments. It is important to distinguish the different phenotypes of WRR, including WER and OR, as this could medicolegally affect the worker. OR is strongly associated with OA, and the early recognition of OR may be an important surveillance marker for future development of OA. When treating patients who present with WRR, the physician should use a detailed history and objective measures, which should include a nasal provocation test if possible. Identifying a causative agent is the primary purpose of an investigation, and eliminating or reducing exposure to the causative agent is of upmost importance. Pharmacologic management should be modeled by current rhinitis therapies. AIT may play a role in treatment, as it has been shown to be effective in treating HMW agents. Further research is needed to better categorize causative agents, identify effective immunosurveillance techniques, and establish effective therapies to reduce the burden of WRR.

REFERENCES

1. Siracusa A, Desrosiers M, Marabini A. Epidemiology of occupational rhinitis: prevalence, aetiology and determinants. Clin Exp Allergy 2000;30(11):1519–34.
2. Moscato G, Vandenplas O, Van Wijk RG, et al. EAACI position paper on occupational rhinitis. Respir Res 2009;10:16.

3. Zeiss CR, Patterson R, Pruzansky JJ, et al. Trimellitic anhydride-induced airway syndromes: clinical and immunologic studies. J Allergy Clin Immunol 1977; 60(2):96–103.

4. Merget R, Kulzer R, Dierkes-Globisch A, et al. Exposure–effect relationship of platinum salt allergy in a catalyst production plant: conclusions from a 5-year prospective cohort study. J Allergy Clin Immunol 2000;105:364–70.

5. Meggs WJ. Hypothesis for induction and propagation of chemical sensitivity based on biopsy studies. Environ Health Perspect 1997;105(Suppl 2):473–8.

6. Castano R, Theriault G. Defining and classifying occupational rhinitis. J Laryngol Otol 2006;120(10):812–7.

7. Ruoppi P, Koistinen T, Susitaival P, et al. Frequency of allergic rhinitis to laboratory animals in university employees as confirmed by chamber challenges. Allergy 2004;59(3):295–301.

8. Jang JH, Kim DW, Kim SW, et al. Allergic rhinitis in laboratory animal workers and its risk factors. Ann Allergy Asthma Immunol 2009;102(5):373–7.

9. Schumacher MJ, Tait BD, Holmes MC. Allergy to murine antigens in a biological research institute. J Allergy Clin Immunol 1981;68(4):310–8.

10. Slovak AJ, Orr RG, Teasdale EL. Efficacy of the helmet respirator in occupational asthma due to laboratory animal allergy (LAA). Am Ind Hyg Assoc J 1985;46(8): 411–5.

11. Nieuwenhuijsen MJ, Putcha V, Gordon S, et al. Exposure–response relations among laboratory animal workers exposed to rats. Occup Environ Med 2003; 60(2):104–8.

12. Heederik D, Venables KM, Malmberg P, et al. Exposure–response relationships for work-related sensitization in workers exposed to rat urinary allergens: results from a pooled study. J Allergy Clin Immunol 1999;103(4):678–84.

13. Renstrom A, Malmberg P, Larsson K, et al. Prospective study of laboratory animal allergy: factors predisposing to sensitization and development of allergic symptoms. Allergy 1994;49(7):548–52.

14. Gautrin D, Ghezzo H, Infante-Rivard C, et al. Incidence and host determinants of work-related rhinoconjunctivitis in apprentice pastry makers. Allergy 2002;57(10): 913–8.

15. Walusiak J, Hanke W, Gorski P, et al. Respiratory allergy in apprentice bakers: do occupational allergies follow the allergic march? Allergy 2004;59(4):442–50.

16. Houba R, Heederik D, Doekes G. Wheat sensitization and work-related symptoms in the baking industry are preventable. An epidemiologic study. Am J Respir Crit Care Med 1998;158:1499–503.

17. Cullinan P, Lowson D, Nieuwenhuijsen MJ, et al. Work related symptoms, sensitisation, and estimated exposure in workers not previously exposed to flour. Occup Environ Med 1994;51(9):579–83.

18. Sander I, Flagge A, Merget R, et al. Identification of wheat flour allergens by means of 2-dimensional immunoblotting. J Allergy Clin Immunol 2001;107(5):907–13.

19. Weichel M, Glaser AG, Ballmer-Weber BK, et al. Wheat and maize thioredoxins: a novel cross-reactive cereal allergen family related to baker's asthma. J Allergy Clin Immunol 2006;117(3):676–81.

20. Bernstein DI, Karnani R, Biagini RE, et al. Clinical and occupational outcomes in health care workers with natural rubber latex allergy. Ann Allergy Asthma Immunol 2003;90(2):209–13.

21. Vandenplas O, Delwiche JP, Depelchin S, et al. Latex gloves with a lower protein content reduce bronchial reactions in subjects with occupational asthma caused by latex. Am J Respir Crit Care Med 1995;151:887–91.

22. Schwartz HJ, Arnold JL, Strohl KP. Occupational allergic rhinitis reaction to psyllium. J Occup Med 1989;31(7):624–6.
23. Vandenplas O, Larbanois A, Vanassche F, et al. Latex-induced occupational asthma: time trend in incidence and relationship with hospital glove policies. Allergy 2009;64(3):415–20.
24. Johnsen CR, Sorensen TB, Ingemann Larsen A, et al. Allergy risk in an enzyme-producing plant: a retrospective follow up study. Occup Environ Med 1997;54(9):671–5.
25. van Rooy FG, Houba R, Palmen N, et al. A cross-sectional study among detergent workers exposed to liquid detergent enzymes. Occup Environ Med 2009;66(11):759–65.
26. Cullinan P, Harris JM, Newman Taylor AJ, et al. An outbreak of asthma in a modern detergent factory. Lancet 2000;356(9245):1899–900.
27. Welinder H, Nielsen J, Bensryd I, et al. IgG antibodies against polyisocyanates in car painters. Clin Allergy 1988;18(1):85–93.
28. Bernstein DI, Korbee L, Stauder T, et al. The low prevalence of occupational asthma and antibody-dependent sensitization to diphenylmethane diisocyanate in a plant engineered for minimal exposure to diisocyanates. J Allergy Clin Immunol 1993;92(3):387–96.
29. Baur X, Marek W, Ammon J, et al. Respiratory and other hazards of isocyanates. Int Arch Occup Environ Health 1994;66(3):141–52.
30. Sari-Minodier I, Charpin D, Signouret M, et al. Prevalence of self-reported respiratory symptoms in workers exposed to isocyanates. J Occup Environ Med 1999;41(7):582–8.
31. Littorin M, Welinder H, Skarping G, et al. Exposure and nasal inflammation in workers heating polyurethane. Int Arch Occup Environ Health 2002;75(7):468–74.
32. Nielsen GD, Olsen O, Larsen ST, et al. IgE-mediated sensitisation, rhinitis and asthma from occupational exposures. Smoking as a model for airborne adjuvants? Toxicology 2005;216:87–105.
33. Siracusa A, Marabini A, Folletti I, et al. Smoking and occupational asthma. Clin Exp Allergy 2006;36(5):577–84.
34. Malo JL, Lemiere C, Desjardins A, et al. Prevalence and intensity of rhinoconjunctivitis in subjects with occupational asthma. Eur Respir J 1997;10(7):1513–5.
35. Karjalainen A, Martikainen R, Klaukka T, et al. Risk of asthma among Finnish patients with occupational rhinitis. Chest 2003;123(1):283–8.
36. Cartier A, Bernstein IL, Burge PS, et al. Guidelines for bronchoprovocation on the investigation of occupational asthma. Report of the Subcommittee on Bronchoprovocation for Occupational Asthma. J Allergy Clin Immunol 1989;84:823–9.
37. Smith AB, Castellan RM, Lewis D, et al. Guidelines for the epidemiologic assessment of occupational asthma. Report of the Subcommittee on the Epidemiologic Assessment of Occupational Asthma, Occupational Lung Disease Committee. J Allergy Clin Immunol 1989;84:794–805.
38. Bernstein JA. Material safety data sheets: are they reliable in identifying human hazards? J Allergy Clin Immunol 2002;110(1):35–8.
39. Howarth PH, Persson CG, Meltzer EO, et al. Objective monitoring of nasal airway inflammation in rhinitis. J Allergy Clin Immunol 2005;115:S414–41.
40. Nathan RA, Eccles R, Howarth PH, et al. Objective monitoring of nasal patency and nasal physiology in rhinitis. J Allergy Clin Immunol 2005;115:S442–59.
41. Hellgren J, Eriksson C, Karlsson G, et al. Nasal symptoms among workers exposed to soft paper dust. Int Arch Occup Environ Health 2001;74(2):129–32.

42. Castano R, Theriault G, Gautrin D, et al. Reproducibility of acoustic rhinometry in the investigation of occupational rhinitis. Am J Rhinol 2007;21(4):474–7.
43. Pepys J, Wells ID, D'Souza MF, et al. Clinical and immunological responses to enzymes of *Bacillus subtilis* in factory workers and consumers. Clin Allergy 1973;3(2):143–60.
44. Grammer LC, Harris KE, Yarnold PR. Effect of respiratory protective devices on development of antibody and occupational asthma to an acid anhydride. Chest 2002;121(4):1317–22.
45. Laoprasert N, Swanson MC, Jones RT, et al. Inhalation challenge testing of latex-sensitive health care workers and the effectiveness of laminar flow HEPA-filtered helmets in reducing rhinoconjunctival and asthmatic reactions. J Allergy Clin Immunol 1998;102:998–1004.
46. Wallace DV, Dykewicz MS, Bernstein DI, et al. The diagnosis and management of rhinitis: an updated practice parameter. J Allergy Clin Immunol 2008;122(Suppl 2): S1–84.
47. Hanrahan LP, Paramore LC. Aeroallergens, allergic rhinitis, and sedating antihistamines: risk factors for traumatic occupational injury and economic impact. Am J Ind Med 2003;44(4):438–46.
48. Walker SM, Pajno GB, Lima MT, et al. Grass pollen immunotherapy for seasonal rhinitis and asthma: a randomized, controlled trial. J Allergy Clin Immunol 2001; 107(1):87–93.
49. Sastre J, Quirce S. Immunotherapy: an option in the management of occupational asthma? Curr Opin Allergy Clin Immunol 2006;6(2):96–100.
50. Armentia A, Martin-Santos JM, Quintero A, et al. Bakers' asthma: prevalence and evaluation of immunotherapy with a wheat flour extract. Ann Allergy 1990;65(4): 265–72.

Index

Note: Page numbers of article titles are in **boldface** type.

A

Acid anhydride chemicals, asthma due to, 669
Acoustic rhinometry, for rhinitis, 792
Acrylates, asthma due to, 692
Airway, remodeling of, 704, 754
Airway responsiveness, in irritant-induced asthma, 753
Airway sensory hyperreactivity, 756
Alendronate, asthma due to, 690
Allergen(s). *See also* Animal allergens.
    in irritant-induced asthma, 753
Allergen immunotherapy, for rhinitis, 793
Allergic occupational rhinitis, 787–788
Allergy, definition of, 748–749
Aluminum production, potroom asthma in, 648–650, 756
Amblyseius californicus, asthma due to, 689
American Thoracic Society, work-exacerbated asthma definition of, 655
5-Aminosalicylic acid, asthma due to, 690
Animal allergens
    asthma due to, 667, 689
    hypersensitivity pneumonitis due to, 770–771
    rhinitis due to, 789–790
Antihistamines, for rhinitis, 793
Antioxidants, 707
Ardystil syndrome, 781
Aspergillus, enzymes derived from, asthma due to, 682
Asthma, work-related. *See* Occupational asthma; Work-related asthma.
Asthmalike disorders, definition of, 649–650
Avoidance
    for hypersensitivity pneumonitis, 782
    for rhinitis, 782–793

B

Bakers
    asthma in, 667, 683, 687–688
    rhinitis in, 790
Beclomethasone, for hypersensitivity pneumonitis, 782
Berylliosis, 779
Biopsy, for hypersensitivity pneumonitis, 778–779
Bird raising industry, hypersensitivity pneumonitis in, 770–771
Bovine serum albumin powder, asthma due to, 689
Breathing pattern, in irritant-induced asthma, 752

Immunol Allergy Clin N Am 31 (2011) 797–805
doi:10.1016/S0889-8561(11)00098-1
0889-8561/11/$ – see front matter © 2011 Elsevier Inc. All rights reserved.
immunology.theclinics.com

United States Postal Service

Statement of Ownership, Management, and Circulation
(All Periodicals Publications Except Requestor Publications)

1. Publication Title	2. Publication Number	3. Filing Date
Immunology and Allergy Clinics of North America	0 0 6 - 3 6 1	9/16/11

4. Issue Frequency	5. Number of Issues Published Annually	6. Annual Subscription Price
Feb, May, Aug, Nov	4	$272.00

7. Complete Mailing Address of Known Office of Publication (Not printer) (Street, city, county, state, and ZIP+4®)

Elsevier Inc.
360 Park Avenue South
New York, NY 10010-1710

Contact Person
Stephen Bushing

Telephone (Include area code)
215-239-3688

8. Complete Mailing Address of Headquarters or General Business Office of Publisher (Not printer)

Elsevier Inc., 360 Park Avenue South, New York, NY 10010-1710

9. Full Names and Complete Mailing Addresses of Publisher, Editor, and Managing Editor (Do not leave blank)

Publisher (Name and complete mailing address)

Kim Murphy, Elsevier, Inc., 1600 John F. Kennedy Blvd. Suite 1800, Philadelphia, PA 19103-2899

Editor (Name and complete mailing address)

Rachel Glover, Elsevier, Inc., 1600 John F. Kennedy Blvd. Suite 1800, Philadelphia, PA 19103-2899

Managing Editor (Name and complete mailing address)

Sarah Barth, Elsevier, Inc., 1600 John F. Kennedy Blvd. Suite 1800, Philadelphia, PA 19103-2899

10. Owner (Do not leave blank. If the publication is owned by a corporation, give the name and address of the corporation immediately followed by the names and addresses of all stockholders owning or holding 1 percent or more of the total amount of stock. If not owned by a corporation, give the names and addresses of the individual owners. If owned by a partnership or other unincorporated firm, give its name and address as well as those of each individual owner. If the publication is published by a nonprofit organization, give its name and address.)

Full Name	Complete Mailing Address
Wholly owned subsidiary of	4520 East-West Highway
Reed/Elsevier, US holdings	Bethesda, MD 20814

11. Known Bondholders, Mortgagees, and Other Security Holders Owning or Holding 1 Percent or More of Total Amount of Bonds, Mortgages, or Other Securities. If none, check box ☐ None

Full Name	Complete Mailing Address
N/A	

12. Tax Status (For completion by nonprofit organizations authorized to mail at nonprofit rates) (Check one)
The purpose, function, and nonprofit status of this organization and the exempt status for federal income tax purposes:
☐ Has Not Changed During Preceding 12 Months
☐ Has Changed During Preceding 12 Months (Publisher must submit explanation of change with this statement)

PS Form 3526, September 2007 (Page 1 of 3 (Instructions Page 3)) PSN 7530-01-000-9931 PRIVACY NOTICE: See our Privacy policy in www.usps.com

---

13. Publication Title	14. Issue Date for Circulation Data Below
Immunology and Allergy Clinics of North America	August 2011

15. Extent and Nature of Circulation		Average No. Copies Each Issue During Preceding 12 Months	No. Copies of Single Issue Published Nearest to Filing Date
a. Total Number of Copies (Net press run)		851	672
b. Paid Circulation (By Mail and Outside the Mail)	(1) Mailed Outside-County Paid Subscriptions Stated on PS Form 3541. (Include paid distribution above nominal rate, advertiser's proof copies, and exchange copies)	366	329
	(2) Mailed In-County Paid Subscriptions Stated on PS Form 3541 (Include paid distribution above nominal rate, advertiser's proof copies, and exchange copies)		
	(3) Paid Distribution Outside the Mails Including Sales Through Dealers and Carriers, Street Vendors, Counter Sales, and Other Paid Distribution Outside USPS®	119	82
	(4) Paid Distribution by Other Classes Mailed Through the USPS (e.g. First-Class Mail®)		
c. Total Paid Distribution (Sum of 15b (1), (2), (3), and (4))	▶	485	411
d. Free or Nominal Rate Distribution (By Mail and Outside the Mail)	(1) Free or Nominal Rate Outside-County Copies Included on PS Form 3541	62	61
	(2) Free or Nominal Rate In-County Copies Included on PS Form 3541		
	(3) Free or Nominal Rate Copies Mailed at Other Classes Through the USPS (e.g. First-Class Mail)		
	(4) Free or Nominal Rate Distribution Outside the Mail (Carriers or other means)		
e. Total Free or Nominal Rate Distribution (Sum of 15d (1), (2), (3) and (4))	▶	62	61
f. Total Distribution (Sum of 15c and 15e)	▶	547	472
g. Copies not Distributed (See instructions to publishers #4 (page #3))	▶	304	200
h. Total (Sum of 15f and g)	▶	851	672
i. Percent Paid (15c divided by 15f times 100)		88.67%	87.08%

16. Publication of Statement of Ownership
If the publication is a general publication, publication of this statement is required. Will be printed in the **November 2011** issue of this publication.
☐ Publication not required

17. Signature and Title of Editor, Publisher, Business Manager, or Owner

Stephen R. Bushing
Stephen R. Bushing -Inventory/Distribution Coordinator

Date
September 16, 2011

I certify that all information furnished on this form is true and complete. I understand that anyone who furnishes false or misleading information on this form or who omits material or information requested on the form may be subject to criminal sanctions (including fines and imprisonment) and/or civil sanctions (including civil penalties).

PS Form 3526, September 2007 (Page 2 of 3)

Moving?

Make sure your subscription moves with you!

To notify us of your new address, find your **Clinics Account Number** (located on your mailing label above your name), and contact customer service at:

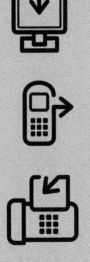

Email: journalscustomerservice-usa@elsevier.com

800-654-2452 (subscribers in the U.S. & Canada)
314-447-8871 (subscribers outside of the U.S. & Canada)

Fax number: 314-447-8029

Elsevier Health Sciences Division
Subscription Customer Service
3251 Riverport Lane
Maryland Heights, MO 63043

ELSEVIER

Printed and bound by CPI Group (UK) Ltd, Croydon, CR0 4YY

03/10/2024

01040447-0017